Joaquim Alves Diniz
Poliana M M de Carvalho
Cleberton Torres Santos

Potentially Inappropriate Medicines for the Elderly

Joaquim Alves Diniz
Poliana M M de Carvalho
Cleberton Torres Santos

Potentially Inappropriate Medicines for the Elderly

In Geriatric Prescriptions

ScienciaScripts

Imprint

Any brand names and product names mentioned in this book are subject to trademark, brand or patent protection and are trademarks or registered trademarks of their respective holders. The use of brand names, product names, common names, trade names, product descriptions etc. even without a particular marking in this work is in no way to be construed to mean that such names may be regarded as unrestricted in respect of trademark and brand protection legislation and could thus be used by anyone.

Cover image: www.ingimage.com

This book is a translation from the original published under ISBN 978-613-9-61690-9.

Publisher:
Sciencia Scripts
is a trademark of
Dodo Books Indian Ocean Ltd. and OmniScriptum S.R.L publishing group

120 High Road, East Finchley, London, N2 9ED, United Kingdom
Str. Armeneasca 28/1, office 1, Chisinau MD-2012, Republic of Moldova, Europe
Printed at: see last page
ISBN: 978-620-7-89051-4

Table of contents:

JOAQUIM ALVES DINIZ
POLIANA MOREIRA MEDEIROS DE CARVALHO
CLEBERTON TORRES SANTOS
ELIANI DA SILVA FREITAS

PHARMACEUTICAL ANALYSIS OF POTENTIALLY INAPPROPRIATE DRUGS IN GERIATRIC PRESCRIPTIONS JUAZEIRO DO NORTE-CE
2018

SUMMARY

The aging process is marked by a greater number of chronic degenerative diseases, which predisposes the geriatric population to be treated with a greater number of drugs, thus increasing the risks related to therapy, such as adverse reactions and drug interactions. This is a descriptive, cross-sectional study based on retrospective analysis of medical prescriptions for individuals aged 60 and over (n=50), drawn up between January and December 2017. Sociodemographic, clinical and pharmacotherapy variables of the elderly were analyzed. The drugs prescribed were categorized according to the Brazilian Consensus on PIM (2016), whose prescriptions should be avoided regardless of clinical condition. There was a predominance of males (58%, n=28/50). The average age was between 70-79 years (40%). The main medical diagnoses were: Systemic Arterial Hypertension (96%); Diabetes *Mellitus (*52%); Dyslipidemia (38%); Osteoporosis (28%) and Depression (24%). Polypharmacy was 56% (n=28/50) among the elderly who used 3 to 5 drugs. Drugs that act on the Central Nervous System (28%), followed by those that act on the Cardiovascular System (26%) were the most prescribed. The most prescribed PIMs were Omeprazole (76%); Amitriptyline (14%); Diazepam (10%) and Glibenclamide (18%). Drug interactions were obtained using Micromedex® Solutions 2018 software. There was a prevalence of 24 moderate and 19 major interactions. The data obtained in this study was relevant in the context of public health, as it revealed important variables relating to knowledge of the pharmacoepidemiology of potentially inappropriate medicines for the elderly. Highlighting the risks of using PIMs in the elderly, as was done in this study, demonstrates that pharmaceutical interventions should be carried out in the context of multidisciplinary care to guarantee access to safe medicines that are appropriate to the specificities of the elderly's pharmacotherapy.

Keywords: Potentially Inappropriate Medications in the Elderly. Pharmaceutical Care in Geriatrics. Geriatric pharmacoepidemiology.

Chapter 1

1 INTRODUCTION

Prospective data from the World Health Organization (WHO, 2015) estimate that by the year 2050, Brazil will experience important demographic changes, in which the elderly population will rise from the current 12.5% to approximately 30%, accentuating what is called population aging (CRUZ *et al*; 2017).

Torres *et al*; (2015), consider that the longer life of human beings is the result of factors such as nutrition, improved health conditions, advances in diagnostic medicine and drugs. Pereira (2016) adds that the decrease in infant mortality and the fertility rate are factors that have accentuated the ageing of the population.

The increase in longevity has also contributed to changes in the epidemiological profile of the world's and Brazil's population, leading to a higher prevalence of chronic non-communicable diseases (CNCDs), such as Systemic Arterial Hypertension (SAH), Diabetes *Mellitus* and Dyslipidemia, which require continuous treatment (MINISTÉRIO DA SAÚDE, 2014).

Lutz, Miranda and Bertoldi (2017) point out that the physiological changes resulting from the ageing process considerably affect the pharmacokinetics and pharmacodynamics of medicines in the elderly. Becerra *et al*; (2015) point out that polypharmacy is a conditioning factor for the increased incidence of adverse drug reactions (ADRs), as well as drug interactions.

In general, the elderly consume an average of between two and five medicines a day, which at some point leads to the use of Potentially Inappropriate Medicines (PIMs), which generate avoidable problems such as colds, falls, depression, hip fractures, immobility and mental confusion (VRDOLJAK and BOROVAC, 2015).

In this context, the multidisciplinary work of the health team is to prevent the most typical syndromes in the elderly: Cognitive incapacity, Postural instability, Immobility, Sphincteric incontinence, Iatrogeny, Communication incapacity and Family insufficiency (CONCEIQÁO, SARRAF and PINHEIRO, 2016).

Santos and Cunha (2017) emphasize that polypharmacy predisposes the elderly population to risks of exposure to the prescription of PIMs, which constitutes a field of intervention for pharmaceutical care, in which the evaluation of pharmacotherapy becomes indispensable. (ESTEVE, *et al*; 2017).

Fastbom and Johnell (2015), Hilário *et al;* (2015) report that inadequate prescribing for the elderly has become a public health issue, due to the morbidity, mortality and hospitalizations caused by the use of PIMs.

The appropriateness of prescribing medication for the elderly is not simple, as it involves several factors that impact on the choice of the correct, safe and effective medication, such as the health situation of the elderly person and aspects involving the pharmacokinetics and pharmacodynamics of the medication (MALAQUIAS *et al*; 2016).

According to this line of reasoning, clinical criteria have been developed to help improve the quality and safety of drug prescriptions for the elderly (VÁSQUEZ, SAAVEDRA and MONTENEGRO, 2016). The Beers-Fick criteria; Screening Tool of Older Person's Prescriptions (STOPP) and Screening Tool to Alert doctors to Right Treatment (START) are the most widely referenced in the literature (GARCÍA *et al*; 2016).

Manso *et al;* (2015), mentioning these criteria, argue that in view of the differences in the availability of medicines, as well as the different prescriptive behaviors, these instruments have been adapted in various countries.

In Brazil, in 2016, the first Brazilian Consensus of Potentially Inappropriate Medicines for the Elderly was published, validated based on the 2012 Beers Criteria and the 2006 STOPP, the final draft of which resulted in a national list of criteria for classifying PIMs, which in fact contributes to better guidance for health professionals in caring for elderly patients (OLIVEIRA, *et al,* 2016).

In this situational framework, it is considered from the reading of Andrade, Silva Filho and Junqueira (2016), that the aging process affects the patient's therapeutic response, which makes prescribing medications a challenge for prescribing professionals.

Lutz, Miranda and Bertoldi (2017) state that the presence of a multidisciplinary team, which includes the pharmacist, will become an indispensable component in the evaluation of pharmacotherapy, because, although polypharmacotherapy is in some cases justified by clinical evidence or therapeutic protocols, there is a need to evaluate the risks/benefits of prescribing (ANDRADE *et al;* 2016).

Chapter 2

2 PROBLEM

The Ministry of Health (2010), through the National Health Promotion Policy, has recommended that the various programs of the Unified Health System (SUS), especially those of the Family Health Strategy (ESF), take action to control CNCDs, in which incentives for healthy lifestyle habits are considered priorities.

However, data from the National Health Survey (2013) show that an average of 60 million Brazilians are affected by at least one NCD, and that the elderly population makes up a large part of this group, and that in order to control NCDs, they make chronic use of medication (IBGE, 2013).

Pharmaceutical Assistance, a public policy that guarantees access to essential medicines, is also involved in the context of the National Health Promotion Policy, as it must guarantee the rational prescription and use of medicines, avoiding undesirable clinical situations due to the inappropriate use of medicines.

As medication is the main therapeutic means for controlling CNCDs, scientific evidence has shown that the use of PIMs is related to undesirable clinical outcomes, which could be avoided due to the existence of safer alternatives for elderly patients (SANTO and CUNHA, 2017; LUTZ, MIRANDA and BERTOLDI, 2017; VÁSQUEZ *et al*, 2016; RODRIGUES and OLIVEIRA, 2016).

In this context, the research problem arises from the identification that the planning of Pharmaceutical Care and medical protocols for the control of NCDs in the elderly are indispensable requirements to avoid the inappropriate use of medicines.

This issue is of great clinical relevance, especially in the elderly population, due to the following factors: the progressive increase in the number of elderly people in Brazil; the high prevalence of multiple CNCDs, polypharmacy, as well as the interference of physiological changes in the pharmacokinetic and pharmacodynamic process, increasing the risk of drug toxicity.

Chapter 3

3 BACKGROUND

The distribution profile of the Brazilian age pyramid has shown serious changes due to the increase in the number of elderly people in the total population, which means that there will be a simultaneous increase in the frequency of hospital admissions, due to the higher prevalence of CNCDs and the greater consumption of medicines (IBGE, 2010).

The elderly have pharmacokinetic and pharmacodynamic characteristics that make them particularly vulnerable to adverse effects (LUTZ, MIRANDA AND BERTOLDI, 2017). Thus, drugs considered inappropriate should be avoided in these patients, as the adverse effects outweigh the clinical benefit. (MUNIZ *et al*; 2017).

Despite the existence of potentially inappropriate drugs in the elderly, explicit criteria are used to determine the appropriateness of pharmacological treatments and protocols are in place to detect potentially inappropriate prescriptions. Among the most widely used are the Beers, STOPP and START criteria (GARCÍA *et al*; 2016).

Considering that medical prescriptions in the SUS, especially those from the ESF, are established according to the list authorized by REMUNE, verifying the presence of MPI, as well as the existence of safe therapeutic alternatives, becomes a critical need in the context of public health.

In this context, and given the changes related to the ageing of the Brazilian population, it is necessary to know the profile of the diseases that affect them and the use of medicines by this population, so that strategies can be established for rational prescribing, avoiding damage to the health of the elderly due to the inappropriate use of medicines.

For the study, the list standardized by the Brazilian Consensus of Potentially Inappropriate Medicines for the Elderly (2016) was used as a parameter for quantitative analysis of the possible clinical findings resulting from the use of PIMs in the prescriptions of elderly patients.

Chapter 4

4 GENERAL OBJECTIVE

To map the prescription of potentially inappropriate medicines (PIM) described in the medical records of elderly patients at a family health strategy unit in Juazeiro do Norte, Ceará.

4.1 Specific objectives

5. Estimate the prevalence of polypharmacy in the elderly (polypharmacy is considered to be the simultaneous use of 3 or more drugs);

6. Analyze the occurrence of problems related to the selection and prescribing of potentially inappropriate medication in the elderly;

7. To estimate the prevalence of potentially inappropriate medications for the elderly according to the criteria of the Brazilian Consensus;

Chapter 5

5 THEORETICAL FRAMEWORK

5.1 GERIATRIC PHARMACOEPIDEMIOLOGY

Aspects related to the ageing of the population are considered a worldwide phenomenon, and are one of the greatest challenges for public health, and Brazil is part of this situation (SANTOS and CUNHA, 2017).

According to 2010 census data from the Brazilian Institute of Geography and Statistics (IBGE), the elderly make up 10.7% (approximately 19 million people) of the Brazilian population, making it a structurally ageing country (IBGE, 2010).

The same data also projects that Brazil's elderly population will total 30 million by 2020, which will represent an average of 13% of the population (IBGE, 2010).

Salech, Palma and Garrido (2016) consider that the increase in life expectancy is mainly due to public health actions, such as vaccinations, access to essential medicines, basic sanitation, and medical and technological advances, which have contributed to a better quality of life.

Associated with longer life expectancy and consequently the increase in the elderly population, the demands for attention and care are also increasing, since the elderly have a higher prevalence of CNCDs, a decline in functional capacity and less autonomy (SILVA *et al*; 2016).

According to data confirmed in 2013 by the National Health Survey (PNS), the elderly have the highest number of CNCDs, such as Diabetes *Mellitus*, Systemic Arterial Hypertension (SAH) and Dyslipidemia. A previous study by Silva *et al;* (2012), revealed that 80% of elderly Brazilians are affected by one or more NCDs and 36% may be affected by three of them.

The study by Goulart *et al.* (2014) found that 44.88% (n=114) of the elderly under analysis had diseases related to the circulatory system (prevalence of 87.72% for hypertension and 9.65% for heart disease), followed by 21.65% for endocrine, nutritional and metabolic disorders and 12.60 for diseases related to the muscular system and connective tissue.

Cobas *et al;* (2017), point out that due to the prevalence of NCDs in the elderly, they are exposed to multiple medications, and that the majority consume at least one and about a third of them are multi-users, consuming five or more simultaneously, a practice conceptualized as polypharmacy. Another population-based study of 934 elderly people in Goiania, Brazil, found an average consumption of 3.63 medicines/elderly person, with a prevalence of polypharmacy of 26.4% (SANTOS *et al*; 2013).

Based on what Andrade, Filho and Junqueira (2016) say, polypharmacy is a common practice among the elderly, and correlates with the following factors: female gender, hospitalization, consultations with different prescribers, self-medication, low perception of health and quality of life.

Santos and Cunha (2017) carried out an important cross-sectional study with 340 individuals aged 60 or over, looking at the factors associated with medication consumption among the elderly in a basic health unit. In this study, a prevalence of 99.7% of medication use was identified and 35.3% used polypharmacotherapy.

Manso, Biffi and Gerard (2015) consider that the use of multiple medications has had a negative impact on the health of the elderly, especially when related to those that are potentially inappropriate.

Relevant factors in this damage are physiological changes that modify pharmacodynamics and pharmacokinetics, contributing to drug toxicity (MASCARENHAS *et al*; 2014).

The literature presents polypharmacy as the practice of using three or more drugs simultaneously, which can result in adverse reactions, interactions and the use of inappropriate treatments (LINJAKUMPU *et al.*, 2002; FLORES; MENGUE, 2005; GORARD, 2006; MEDEIROS, 2007; DAL PIZZOL, 2012).

Andrade, Filho and Junqueira (2016) add that polypharmacy predisposes to drug iatrogenesis, which occurs when a drug causes a pathogenic effect in isolation or through the interaction of several drugs. These factors ultimately lead to drug intoxication.

In relation to studies on the use of medicines in the elderly, the analysis by Santos and Cunha (2017) correlated the use of antihypertensives, diuretics and antidiabetics as the most prescribed. The table below summarizes important Brazilian studies that list the main pharmacological classes prescribed to the elderly.

Most prescribed pharmacological classes	Type of study	References
Antihypertensives (75 %) **Analgesics-antiflammatories (60%)** **Diuretics (53.2%)** **Antidiabetics (38.5%) Lipid-lowering agents (34.10%)**	A cross-sectional study of 340 elderly people aged 60 or over, carried out in 2013, in Sao Paulo, SP.	Santos, cunha (2017). Factors associated with the consumption of medicines between elderly people in a basic health unit
Antihypertensives (8.10%) **Vitamins (8.9%)** **Analgesics (5.54%)**	Cross-sectional and descriptive study carried out with 239 elderly users of supplementary health insurance in a medium-sized municipality in the state of Sao Paulo, Brazil.	Muniz, et al (2017). Analysis of medication use by elderly supplementary health plan users.
Antihypertensives (50.09%) **Anti-inflammatory and anti-rheumatic drugs (82.69%)** **Antidiabetics (53.33%)**	A prospective, cross-sectional study was carried out to assess the profile of consumption medicines by elderly in a ubs in the municipality of Rondonópolis/MT.	Goulart, et al (2014) consumption of medications by the elderly in a basic health unit from Rondonópolis/MT
Antihypertensives (19.7%) **Analgesics-antiflammatories (9.1%)** **Vitamins, supplements, tonics and appetite stimulants, (6.7%)**	Base study population cross-sectional study with 934 elderly people from Goiania, GO, Brazil, between December 2009 and April 2010.	Santos, et al (2013). Consumption medicines by seniors, Goiania, Brazil

Chart 01 - National studies on the prevalence of medication use in the elderly.
Source: Prepared by the author, 2018.

Analysis of the aforementioned pharmacoepidemiological studies indicates that the class of antihypertensive drugs are the most commonly prescribed in elderly patients, due to the fact that diseases of the cardiovascular system, such as SAH, are more prevalent in this population.

Another therapeutic class that deserves attention is anti-inflammatory drugs. The consumption of these drugs tends to occupy a prominent place among the elderly, considering that their consumption is related to the treatment of pain and inflammation, typical symptoms at this stage (CASCAES, FALCHETTI and GALATO, 2008).

In this context, the use of medication by the elderly has a fine line between risk and benefit, that is, the high use of medication can affect the quality of life of the elderly, so it is necessary to establish criteria for the selection of medications that are safe, effective and meet the needs of the elderly population (RODRIGUES and OLIVEIRA, 2016).

Chapter 6

6 PHYSIOLOGICAL ASPECTS OF AGING THAT IMPACT DRUG THERAPY

Nowadays, studies related to the aging process are gaining considerable interest from the perspective of identifying the factors that most influence healthy aging, that is, the reasons that lead some individuals to age with a preserved quality of life (PARENTE, 2016).

Considering that aging is an irreversible process inherent to the human being, Tavares *et al;* (2015), identified that senescence, considered to be the individual's natural aging process, is influenced by environmental factors, such as lifestyle, eating habits and genetics. These are considered key to healthy ageing.

In this context, aging is considered to be a complex and multifaceted biological process due to the occurrence of various physiological changes, which permeate from the tissue level to the organism as a whole (RODRIGUES and OLIVEIRA, 2016).

According to the World Report on Ageing and Health, written by the WHO (2015), the ageing process involves intense and variable molecular and cellular damage which, over time, leads to a gradual loss of physiological reserves, making people susceptible to various diseases.

Chaimowicz (2014) correlates that in addition to the biological changes that occur in the elderly, aging is also influenced by sociodemographic and social variables, which leads to some limitations, making them more susceptible to various illnesses, a factor that contributes to a reduction in quality of life.

Studies have already shown that biological changes occur in the biochemical composition of tissues; there is a progressive decrease in physiological capacity and an increase in susceptibility and vulnerability to diseases (BALDONI *et al,* 2014). Sanche, Gardenghi (2016), consider that psychological and cognitive changes, loss of muscle mass, bone and motor flexibility are physiological changes that also accompany aging.

Gomes *et al.* (2017) point out that in the elderly, the main physiological changes occur in the cardiovascular, nervous and musculoskeletal systems. At the level of the nervous system, the main alteration occurs due to a decrease in brain activity, leading to a decrease in reflexes and sensitivity, a decrease in intellectual capacity and alterations in attention (LINO, 2015).

According to Abreu (2014), changes in the digestive system are one of the main changes related to senescence. In this system, changes such as a reduction in the mechanical and chemical processes of ingestion, digestion and absorption, impaired absorption of nutrients, constipation and a reduction in the half-life of drugs are among the most common.

Pharmacotherapy in these patients is also affected, which requires special care, given the peculiarities presented in pharmacokinetic and pharmacodynamic parameters (MASCARENHAS *et al*; 2014).

On this subject, Salech, Palma and Garrido (2016) described the main physiological events associated with aging, systematized in the following aspects: body composition, absorption, distribution, metabolism and renal function, systematized in the table below.

Chart 02 - Physiological events associated with ageing that have an impact on the pharmacokinetics of medicines.

Body composition	Physiological changes
Body fat	Increased
Lean body mass	Decreased
Body water	Decreased
Absorption	**Physiological changes**
Gastric pH	Increased
Secretory capacity	Decreased
Gastrointestinal blood flow	Decreased
Distribution	**Physiological changes**
Plasma albumin	Decreased
Affinity for proteins	Decreased
al - acid glycoprotein	Increased
Metabolism	**Physiological changes**

Liver size	Decrease
Hepatic blood flow	Decrease
Renal function	**Physiological changes**
Glomerular filtration rate	Decrease
Renal plasma flow	Decrease

Source: Adapted from Salech, Palma and Garrido (2016).

O'Mahony *et al;* (2015), discussing pharmacokinetic aspects in aging, postulate that the absorption of drugs in the elderly may be reduced, since with the decrease in acid production in the stomach, there is a delay in the motility of the digestive tract, which considerably affects the speed and time of gastric emptying.

Drug metabolism is also altered in the elderly. Alecrim *et al*; (2016), state that due to the decrease in hepatic blood flow, drugs can have a prolonged half-life, which can alter the bioavailability of those that undergo first-pass metabolism.

In the elderly, liver function is diminished, not only due to the deficit in blood flow but also due to the loss of muscle mass, a decrease in albumin and hemoglobin levels and an increase in bilirubin levels (TEIXEIRA, 2015).

In the elderly, there is also a decrease in renal flow and glomerular filtration; therefore, when drugs are excreted through the kidneys, there can be an increase in their half-life, which can result in accumulation and toxicity (CUENTRO, *et al.*, 2014).

Another important factor is drug distribution. In the elderly, there is a decrease in albumin levels and an increase in a1-acid glycoprotein, so drug monitoring is necessary. In the case of albumin, there is a decrease in its levels, so it is necessary to reduce the dose administered in view of the greater fraction of free drug, which has a direct impact on plasma bioavailability (GOODMAN, 2006).

In this context, it is correct to say that the decrease in physiological functions in the elderly is considered one of the factors that directly interferes with the pharmacokinetics and pharmacodynamics of drugs, which reinforces the idea that the evaluation of pharmacotherapy in these patients must be careful and specific (GARSKE *et al*; 2016).

6.1 Pharmacological Characterization of Potentially Inappropriate Medications in the Elderly

Pharmacology in the elderly has its own peculiarities, with pharmacokinetic parameters being the main changes affecting the therapeutic response to drugs (SALES, SALES and CASOTTI, 2017).

Dantas (2016) considers that although the control and treatment of most diseases are linked to the use of drug therapy, it is necessary to consider that in the elderly, pharmacotherapy has particularities that can somehow contribute to adverse reactions, including those characterized as iatrogenic.

It should also be borne in mind that, while there are no completely safe drugs, since all of them, in greater or lesser doses, can generate an ADR, in the treatment of the elderly these reactions are potentially more frequent and can expose them to this risk (SANTOS *et al*; 2016).

Lima *et al*; (2016), state that drugs called inappropriate for the elderly are established by expert consensus, such as the Beers-Fick, STOOP, START and PRISCO specifications. However, concerns about the use of drugs for the elderly cannot be restricted to their classification as appropriate or inappropriate, although this is important to mitigate ADRs.

In this context, the Brazilian Consensus on Potentially Inappropriate Medications for the Elderly (2016), considers an inappropriate medication prescription in the following situations:

> *S* Increased risk of ADR when there is evidence of an equally or more effective alternative with lower risk to treat the same clinical condition;
>
> *S* Use of medication with a higher dosage and treatment time than clinically indicated;
>
> *S* Use of multiple medications that have drug or drug-disease interactions;
>
> s Underuse of beneficial drugs that are clinically indicated but not prescribed due to age discrimination or illogical reasons.

As a way of standardizing which medications are considered inappropriate, the Brazilian consensus (2016) systematized them into two conditions: prescriptions that should be avoided regardless of the clinical condition and those that should be avoided taking into account the clinical conditions and diseases of the elderly patient (OLIVEIRA *et al*; 2016).

The adaptability of the list of inappropriate medicines to the Brazilian reality reinforced the idea of how necessary it was to establish these criteria to remedy the differences in prescriptive clinical practice when guided by the Beers and STOPP criteria already consolidated in the literature (CORRÊA, RODRIGUES and MACEDO, 2016).

Sonnichsen *et al,* (2016), consider that avoiding the use of PIMs in the elderly contributes to public health aspects, as it optimizes appropriate prescribing and reduces negative clinical outcomes such as hospitalizations due to preventable ADRs, disability and death.

Chapter 7

7 ACCESS TO ESSENTIAL MEDICINES IN FAMILY HEALTH STRATEGY UNITS

The National Primary Care Policy (PNAB), especially the Family Health Strategy (ESF), is an important space for collective and individual interventions, covering health promotion, prevention, treatment, diagnosis and rehabilitation, with primary care being the user's main gateway to the services of the Unified Health System (SUS) (MINISTÉRIO DA SAÚDE, PNAB, 2012).

Few countries in the world have a system of free health services. Brazil is one of those that has an integrated public health system, with the availability of medical and hospital care, access to medicines, diagnostic and rehabilitation resources (TAVARES and LIMA, 2017).

Nascimento Junior, *et al*, (2015), recalls the important stimulus that the World Health Organization (WHO) has been giving to countries since the 1970s, when it recommended the adoption of national lists that promote access to essential medicines.

In the context of Brazilian Pharmaceutical Assistance, Law 8080/90, in its 6th article, states that the execution of various actions are included in the scope of action of the SUS, including comprehensive therapeutic assistance, including pharmaceutical assistance (BRASIL, 1990).

Still in the field of Brazilian public policy, the Statute of the Elderly (Brazil, 2003) and the National Health Policy for the Elderly (Brazil, 2006) also advocate that it is the government's responsibility to provide free medicines, especially those for continuous use, as an integral part of care for the elderly (BRASIL, Statute of the Elderly, Law No. 57, of September 23, 2003).

In this context, Brazil has drawn up important public policies in the field of pharmaceutical assistance, with the aim of enabling access to medicines for the population. The National Medicines Policy - PNM (Brazil, 1998) and the National Pharmaceutical Assistance Policy - PNAF (Brazil, 2004) are considered to be decisive public policies for this access (NAKATA and SILVA, 2015).

Data from the latest National Household Sample Survey (PNAD, 2012) revealed that the only way for the low-income population to access medicines is through SUS pharmaceutical assistance programs, which is in line with the assumptions of the PNM and PNAF. (IBGE, 2013). Buenos and Oliveira (2011) found that the majority of elderly Brazilians use the SUS to access medicines.

As recommended by the WHO, the SUS provides the population with medicines included in the National List of Essential Medicines (RENAME), prepared through selection processes, based on technical criteria, scientific evidence, nosological and epidemiological profile (FARIA, *et al,* 2015).

The RENAME is the model for drawing up the State List of Medicines (RESME) and in the municipalities for drawing up the Municipal List of Essential Medicines (REMUNE) (FERREIRA, *et al,* 2016). In its recent update (RENAME-2017), it follows the same systematization as previous versions and is organized into pharmaceutical care blocks, as shown below.

Fig 01- Systematization of the blocks of Pharmaceutical Services.

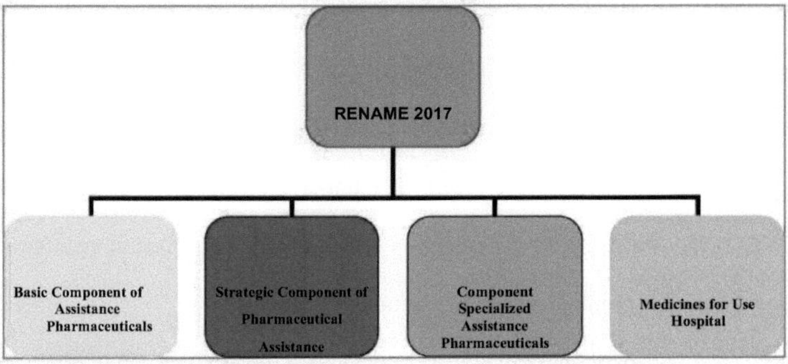

RENAME 2017

Basic Component of Assistance Pharmaceuticals

Strategic Component of Pharmaceutical Assistance

Component Specialized Assistance Pharmaceuticals

Medicines for Use Hospital

Source: Prepared by the author, 2018.

Oliveira, Nascimento and Pereira (2016), consider that the basic component of pharmaceutical care has a very close relationship with most of the demands for drug therapy services within the SUS, as they correspond to the main health problems in primary care that affect the elderly, such as SAH, Diabetes Mellitus and Dyslipidemias.

The pharmaceutical assistance block for primary care is financed by the three federated entities, with municipal management being responsible for the purchase of most medicines and pharmaceutical supplies, with the exception of the purchase and distribution of human insulin (NPH and Regular), oral and injectable contraceptives, intrauterine devices (IUDs) and diaphragms, for which the Ministry of Health is responsible (RENAME, 2017).

Thus, it is clear how important REMUNE is, because it is based on the availability of the medicines on this list that primary care prescribers decide on their therapeutic indication, which in the elderly requires greater care, given the various physiological changes that affect the pharmacokinetics and pharmacodynamics of medicines (CASSONI, *et al,* 2014).

Based on the Beers-2008 methodology, an analysis of REMUNE 2010 in the municipality of Ijuí, RS, Brazil, showed that 15.96% of medicines were considered potentially inappropriate, but that for 86.67% of these there was at least one alternative with a similar indication, which could possibly be used as a substitute (BUENO and OLIVEIRA, 2011).

Another study carried out in 2016 in Ipatinga, MG, Brazil, revealed that of the 245 medicines present in REMUNE, 28 active ingredients are considered potentially inappropriate for the elderly, according to the Beers-Fick 2012 criteria (FERREIRA, et al, 2016).

Diniz, *et al* (2016), analyzing the 2014 version of the STOPP criteria in the RENAME of a municipality in the interior of Ceará, found that of all the 131 medicines dispensed in primary care, 29 active ingredients were considered inappropriate for the elderly. The most prevalent were antihypertensives (9%); drugs that act on the central nervous system (13%) and those with an increased risk of falls in the elderly (benzodiazepines, neuroleptics, antidepressants and 1st generation anti-histamines[a]), corresponding to 23%.

Based on these studies, the fragility of REMUNE is evident when evaluating the group of drugs that are potentially inappropriate for the elderly, which in fact alerts prescribers, pharmacists and nurses to identify such drugs and avoid exposing the elderly to these products as much as possible (FARIA, *et al,* 2015).

Chapter 8

8 RESEARCH METHODOLOGY

This is a descriptive, cross-sectional study whose unit of analysis was the prescription of potentially inappropriate medication for the elderly, collected retrospectively from the medical records of patients assisted at the Family Health Strategy 13 (ESF-13) unit, Antônio Vieira, Juazeiro do Norte/CE.

To carry out a cross-sectional study, the researcher must first define the question to be answered, then define the population to be studied and a method for choosing the sample and, finally, define the phenomena to be studied and the methods for measuring the variables of interest (GIL, 2008).

Therefore, based on the criteria established by the Brazilian Consensus of Potentially Inappropriate Medicines for the Elderly (2016), we investigated whether there were problems related to medicines in the geriatric prescriptions analyzed.

8.1 Inclusion criteria

The sample size was calculated using the following statistical parameters: the elderly population registered at ESF 13 had a total of 219 patients. The sample size was determined using a 95% confidence interval and a 5% sampling error. A minimum of 50 medical records were analyzed and the inclusion criteria were:

-1- age > *60* years;

-2- the prescription was drawn up between January and December 2017;

-3- is written legibly, allowing for complete reading and decoding;

-4- polymedicated elderly (use of 3 or more medications).

8.2 Exclusion criteria

Patients aged 59 or under were excluded from this study, because according to the Statute of the Elderly, a person aged 60 or over is considered elderly (MINISTÉRIO DA SAÚDE. ESTATUTO DO IDOSO, 2003). In addition, the elderly were aged 60 or over and had less than three (3) prescribed medications.

Fig. 02- Flowchart of the Sampling Process

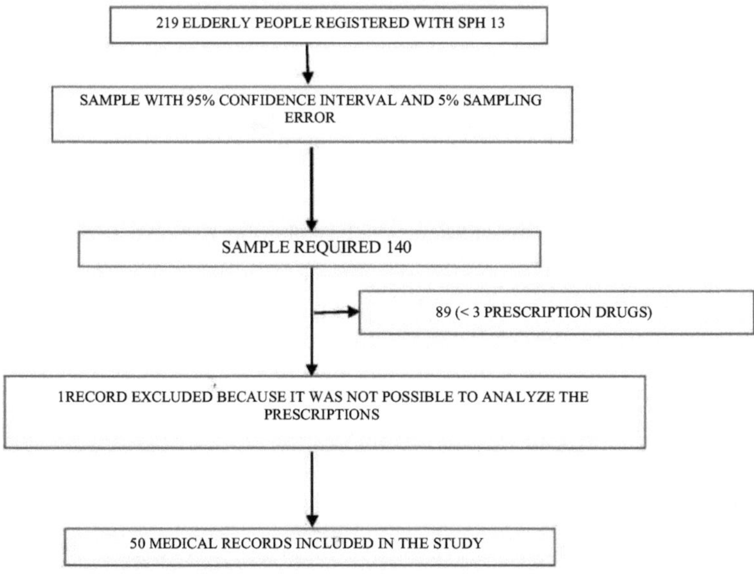

Source: Prepared by the author, 2018.

8.3 Risks

Considering that the data in the medical records is the sole and exclusive property of the patient, who has provided information in a relationship of confidentiality between doctor and patient, in order to carry out their treatment and medical care, and that all research involving human beings involves risks, as dictated by CNS resolution 196/96-V, the risks that could occur are related to the improper handling of medical records that leads to their loss or deterioration with substantial loss of the patient's clinical information.

Therefore, as a way of minimizing these risks, the analysis of medical records was carried out in the health unit itself and under the supervision of the person responsible for keeping the document, as well as inspections at the beginning and end of each analysis.

8.4 Benefits

To make a scientific contribution to studies on the use and utilization of medication in geriatrics, highlighting the importance of observing inappropriate medication in the elderly in clinical practice as a way of minimizing medication-related problems in geriatric groups.

Chapter 9

9 DATA COLLECTION AND TABULATION

Data was collected using forms adapted from the Ministry of Health's standardized forms for pharmaceutical care in primary care, in which the information contained in the patients' records was transcribed, in compliance with the rules of professional secrecy according to CFM Resolution No. 1997/2012.

The forms (Appendix A) were filled in with the following data: sociodemographic variables (gender and age) and clinical variables (diagnosis that led to the prescription; drugs prescribed and prescriber).

9.1 Data tabulation

Descriptive statistics were used to quantify the primary variables collected: sociodemographic data, recorded medical diagnoses and established pharmacotherapy (including active ingredient, dose, pharmaceutical form and dosage).

Based on this data, the number of drugs prescribed by the elderly and prevalent pathologies were quantified according to the *Anatomical-Therapeutic-Clinical* (ATC) classification proposed by the World Health Organization.

. The so-called secondary variables PIM (Potentially Inappropriate Medications) were estimated based on the prevalence of these medications instrumentalized by the criteria established by the Brazilian Consensus on PIM (2016), independent of clinical condition.

Drug interactions between medicines were checked using the Micromedex® Solutions database (2018), which only estimated potential interactions that had good or excellent documentation in relation to existing scientific knowledge about them, as well as the possible impact of this interaction on the patient (Contraindicated, Major and Moderate).

The research complied with the recommendations of Resolution No. 466/2012 of the National Health Council, and was authorized by the Research Ethics Committee of the Faculty of Juazeiro do Norte (FJN) with opinion No. 2.610.151.

Chapter 10

10 RESULTS AND DISCUSSIONS

The sample comprised the medical prescriptions of 50 elderly patients seen at the Family Health Strategy (ESF-13) in the municipality of Juazeiro do Norte/CE, from January to December 2017.

Table 1 shows the age composition of the sample according to the sociodemographic variables and clinical diagnoses assessed. Males predominated in the sample, 56% (28), while females made up 44% (22) of the population studied.

A similar prevalence was found in the studies by Alvim, *et al* (2015), in which 54% of the medical prescriptions made were for male patients. In an analysis by Tavares, *et al* (2016) in which they evaluated free access to medicines for the treatment of chronic diseases in Brazil, they found that men had a prevalence of 51.4% in relation to access to medicines.

The average age comprised patients between 70-79 years old, which represents 40% of the sample, corroborating the studies carried out by Muniz, et al (2017); Andrade, Silva Filho and Junqueira (2017). (Table 1).

Table 1- Characterization of the elderly according to gender, age and clinical diagnosis - ESF 13, Juazeiro do Norte, Ceará, 2018.

	n	%
Sex (n=50)		
Male	28	56,00
Female	22	44,00
Age (years)		
60-69	15	30,00
70-79	20	40,00
80-89	14	28,00
>90	1	2,00
Main clinical diagnoses		
Anxiety	3	6,00
Depression	12	24,00
Diabetes Mellitus	26	52,00
Dyslipidemia	19	38,00
Gastritis	3	6,00
Systemic Arterial Hypertension (SAH)	46	96,00
Hypothyroidism	1	2,00
Heart Failure	3	6,00
Osteoporosis	14	28,00

Source: Prepared by the author, Diniz (2018).

The clinical diagnosis profile revealed that the main diseases affecting the elderly were: Systemic Arterial Hypertension (96%); Diabetes *Mellitus* (52%); Dyslipidemia (38%); Osteoporosis (28%) and Depression (24%). In the study by Ramos, et al (2016), in which they assessed the profile of drug use and its relationship with chronic diseases, they found that this relationship was mainly related to pathologies related to the cardiovascular system, especially Systemic Arterial Hypertension with a prevalence of 66%.

In important studies carried out by (GALATO, SILVA and TIBURCIO, 2010; JARDIM, BARRETO and GIATTI, 2010; CHEHUEN NETO, et al., 2012), they found frequencies of 43.9%, 46.7%, 63.5% and 73% respectively as a diagnosis for hypertension in the elderly.

Oliveira, Nascimento and Pereira (2016) found an absolute frequency of 91 (n=100) diagnoses related to the cardiovascular system, and SAH is the leading cause of morbidity and mortality in individuals aged over 60. Data presented by Malta, et al (2017) revealed that NCDs are responsible for around 70% of all deaths worldwide, with an estimated 38 million deaths annually.

Brazilian data show that AH affects 32.5% (36 million) of adults and more than 60% of the elderly, contributing directly or indirectly to 50% of deaths from cardiovascular disease (SCALA and MACHADO, 2015).

Still in the context of the main pathologies affecting the elderly, Mascarenhas, et al, (2014) found similar results to this study, in which the main diagnoses were hypertension (80%), hypercholesterolemia (24%), arthritis (22%), osteoporosis (18%), diabetes (14%), sleep disorders (12%), labyrinthitis (12%) and cancer (6%).

In this context, it is common for the elderly to suffer from multiple diseases, mainly chronic-degenerative, which can cause limitations and dependence, the most frequent of which are hypertension, diabetes, arthritis, chronic kidney failure, osteoporosis and dementia (GOULART, et al., 2014).

The Brazilian Society of Cardiology (2010) considers SAH to be one of the most important public health problems, due to its high prevalence, low control rate and one of the main risk factors for brain and cardiovascular diseases.

The 7th Brazilian Hypertension Guideline (2017) considers SAH to be a multifactorial clinical condition characterized by sustained elevation of blood pressure levels > 140 and/or 90 mmHg. In situations of poor blood pressure control, SAH is associated with metabolic disorders, functional and/or structural alterations of target organs, and is aggravated by the presence of other risk factors, such as dyslipidemia, abdominal obesity, glucose intolerance and diabetes *mellitus* (MALACHIAS, et al., 2016).

Galato, Silva and Tibúrcio (2010) consider that cardiovascular problems such as hypertension contribute to the practice of polypharmacy, justified by the appearance of other morbidities that require continuous treatment. Thus, the greater occurrence of diseases of the cardiovascular system causes a high use of medication, as was seen during this study.

Another important finding in this study was the significant number of elderly people with depression, 24% (n=50), which is in line with Silva, et al (2016), who states that depression is the most common mental health problem in the elderly, having a negative impact on all aspects of life, and is therefore of great relevance to public health.

Two major groups of illnesses found in this study, SAH and depression, are closely related to the main pharmacological classes of drugs most prescribed, grouped according to the ATC classification, as shown in table 2 below.

Table 2- Group of drugs most commonly prescribed to the elderly according to the Anatomical Therapeutic Chemical (ATC) classification. ESF 13, Juazeiro do Norte/CE, 2018.

	n° Prescribed Medicines	%
ATC classification levels 1 and 2		
A: Digestive system and metabolism (n=6)		**12,00**
A02B Medicinal products for the treatment of peptic ulcer disease	2	4,00
A10 Medicines used for diabetes	4	8,00
C: Cardiovascular System (n=13)		**26,00**
C01 Cardiac glycoside	1	2,00
C01B Antiarrhythmic, classes I and III	1	2,00
C03 Diuretics	2	4,00
C03D Potassium sparing agents	1	2,00

C07 Beta-blockers	2	4,00
C0 Calcium channel blockers	1	2,00
C09 Agents acting on the renin-angiotensin system	3	6,00
C10 Lipid-lowering agents	2	4,00
N: Nervous System (n=14)		**28,00**
N03 Antiepileptic drugs	3	6,00
N04 Antiparkinsonians	2	4,00
N05 Psycholeptics		
N05A Antipsychotics	3	6,00
N05B Anxiolytics	2	4,00
N06A Antidepressants	4	8,00

Source: Prepared by the author, Diniz (2018).

Drugs that act on the Central Nervous System (28%) were the ones that showed the greatest variability in prescribing, with the subgroup of antidepressants (8%) constituting the majority, a similar prevalence was found in the studies carried out by Faraoni, et al (2015) in which most of the drugs analyzed (51.43%) belonged to the nervous, digestive and respiratory systems.

Drugs that act on the cardiovascular system accounted for 26%, of which agents that act on the renin-angiotensin system (6%) were the most used by the elderly.

In the research carried out by Garske, et al (2016), it was reported that drugs that act on the cardiovascular system presented (42.9%), followed by those that acted on the central nervous system (20.9%), which proves that these therapeutic classes are the most used by the elderly.

A similar study, which analyzed the use of medicines by the elderly in a primary health care unit in Divinópolis/MG, showed significantly the same classes of drugs found in this study, considering the second level of the ATC classification, the most frequently prescribed drugs belonged to the class of diuretics (15.1%), and agents with an action on the renin-angiotensin system (14.6%). (OLIVEIRA, et al, 2016).

Table 3 shows the frequency with which the drugs were prescribed. This showed a frequency of (58%) prescriptions for Hydrochlorothiazide; (32%) Captopril; and (30%) Losartan.

Table 3- Distribution of the drugs most often prescribed to the elderly. ESF 13, Juazeiro do Norte/CE, 2018.

Medicines	Prescription Frequency	%
ASA 100 mg	11	22,00
Alendronate+Ca Carbonate	10	20,00
Amitriptyline	7	14,00
Captopril	16	32,00
Glibenclamide	9	18,00
Hydrochlorothiazide	29	58,00
Losartan	15	30,00
Metformin	21	42,00

Omeprazole	38	76,00
Simvastatin	21	42,00

Source: Prepared by the author, Diniz (2018).

Pinto, et al (2014) showed a similar prevalence of drugs most often prescribed to the elderly: Acetylsalicylic acid (ASA) was present in 31 (77.5%) of the prescriptions, followed by Hydrochlorothiazide - 25(62.5%), Simvastatin - 24 (60.0%), Omeprazole - 24 (60.0%), Metformin - 22 (55.0%), Enalapril - 22 (55.0%), Glibenclamide - 11 (27.5%), Captopril - 7 (17.5%).

Although there are conflicting recommendations as to the type of antihypertensive of first choice, the 7th Brazilian Hypertension Guideline (2017) recommends that drug treatment should begin with the prescription of a class of antihypertensive, in which five important classes with proven efficacy in the treatment of SAH and in reducing morbidity and mortality in hypertensive individuals, should be within the best therapeutic choice, namely : diuretics; beta-blockers; angiotensin-converting enzyme (ACE) inhibitors; AT1 receptor blockers; and calcium channel blockers. This justifies the frequency with which the drugs found in this study are the most prescribed (MALACHIAS, et al., 2016).

In particular, hydrochlorothiazide (58%) was the most prescribed drug. Gontijo, et al (2012) found in an important population survey in Minas Gerais, Brazil, that among elderly hypertensive patients taking antihypertensive drugs (n = 283), the class of drugs most frequently used to control the disease was diuretics (68.2%), especially Hydrochlorothiazide.

The pharmacological action of diuretics is initially related to their natriuretic effects, with a decrease in extracellular volume. After four to six weeks, circulating volume practically normalizes and there is a reduction in peripheral vascular resistance (PVR). Studies have shown the therapeutic efficacy of diuretics with a significant reduction in blood pressure and consequently cardiovascular morbidity and mortality (POULTER, PRABHAKARAN and CAULFIELD, 2015).

Therefore, preference should be given to thiazide or similar diuretics (Chlorthalidone, Hydrochlorothiazide and Indapamide) in low doses, as they are gentler and have a longer duration of action (7ª DIRETRIZ BRASILEIRA DE HIPERTENSÃO ARTERIAL).

Omeprazole was the most prescribed drug (76%), this frequency was due to the fact that more than three drugs were used per prescription, being considered in this situation a gastric protector. Hipólito, Rocha and Oliveira (2016), found a prevalence of (65.60%) prescribing Omeprazole in the elderly, of which (29.5%) had no justification for use.

However, pharmacotherapy with Omeprazole is clinically indicated for the treatment of gastroesophageal reflux disease, erosive esophagitis associated with gastroesophageal reflux disease, hypersecretory conditions (Zollenger-Elison syndrome, hypergastrinemia, systemic mastocytosis and multiple endocrine adenoma), peptic ulcers and Helicobacter pylori eradication therapy (SOUZA et al., 2013).

The studies by Lima and Neto Filho (2013) pointed to possible alterations: decreased absorption of vitamins and minerals that are important for the human body, such as vitamin B12, iron, calcium and magnesium, which can lead to anemia, pneumonia and enteric infections.

In the medical records of the elderly people analyzed, it could be seen that the majority had no justification for prescribing Omeprazole, only (6%) had a medical diagnosis of gastritis (table 1), which does not justify the high frequency of prescriptions (76%), as seen in table 3. In this way, it was possible to identify that some medicines were indicated for the elderly without there being a clear correspondence between the disease and the pharmacological action, leading to irrational use of medicines.

When we analyzed the number of medicines used by the elderly, we found that 56% of them used between 3 and 5 medicines, while 44% used between 6 and 10 medicines, a practice considered to be polypharmacy (Table 4). A considerable prevalence was also found in the studies by Ramos, et al (2016) in which 29.0% of the elderly used three or four medicines and 18.0% used at least five.

The higher prevalence of CNCDs in the elderly results in the practice of polypharmacy, which in turn has an impact on safety and quality of life. Even so, it can lead to adverse reactions and drug interactions (VARALLO, COSTA and MASTROIANNI, 2013; OLIVEIRA, et al, 2011).

In the meantime, it is important to note that the risks of drug interactions increase with the increase in the number of drugs prescribed, as can be seen in table 4 below.

Table 4- Relationship between the number of drugs prescribed and the presence of interactions. ESF 13, Juazeiro do Norte/CE, 2018.

number of medicines per prescription	number of elderly people	prescriptio n number	interactions	by	% of drug-drug interactions
From 3 to 5	28 (56%)		23		82,14
From 6 to 10	22 (44%)		20		90,90

Source: Prepared by the author, Diniz (2018).

Elderly patients who used between 6 and 10 drugs had 20 types of interactions per prescription, corresponding to 90.90%. In general, few studies evaluate drug interactions in primary care patients. Even so, in the studies by Pinto, et al (2014) evaluating the clinical impact of drug interactions in prescriptions for elderly hypertensive patients, they identified 169 drug interactions, of which 139 (82.2%) were moderate, 29 (17.2%) severe and 1 (0.6%) mild, totaling 69 different types.

With regard to the number of interactions, the table below shows that ASA accounted for 5 types of moderate interactions, with undesirable clinical effects. In addition to this study, an investigation of elderly hypertensive patients in southern Brazil found that ASA, Enalapril and Hydrochlorothiazide were among the most commonly used drugs and accounted for the main drug interactions of moderate severity (CODAGNONE, GARCIA and SANTA HELENA, 2010). In another important literature review, Silva and Santos (2011) found that ASA was among the main drugs with potential for drug interactions.

Table 5 - Most frequent moderate drug interactions and <u>available</u> scientific evidence. <u>ESF 13, Juazeiro do Norte/CE, 2018.</u>

Moderate interactions*	Prevalence (n=24)	Scientific Evidence	Clinical effects on the patient
Digoxin + Omeprazole	3	Good	It can result in an increased risk of digoxin toxicity (nausea, vomiting, arrhythmias).
Amitriptyline+Carbamazepine	1	Good	It may result in a decrease in the effectiveness of amitriptyline.
Carbamazepine+Hydrochlorothiazide	1	Good	It can result in hyponatremia.
Carbamazepine+Omeprazole	1	Good	It may result in an increased risk of carbamazepine toxicity.

Enalapril+Ibuprofen	1	Excellent	May result in kidney dysfunction and/or increased blood pressure.
Glibenclamide+Propranolol	1	Good	May result in hypoglycemia or hyperglycemia; decreased symptoms of hypoglycemia.
			May result in hypoglycemia or hyperglycemia; decreased
Metformin+Propranolol	2	Good	symptoms of hypoglycemia. It can result in decreased
Levothyroxine+Omeprazole	2	Good	effectiveness of levothyroxine. May decrease the effectiveness of
Levothyroxine+Sinvastatin	1	Good	levothyroxine. It can result in the loss of
Phenytoin+Sinvastatin	1	Good	effectiveness of simvastatin. May result in decreased
ASA 100 mg+ Captopril	2	Excellent	effectiveness of captopril. May result in decreased

ASA 100 mg+ Enalapril	1	Excellent	effectiveness of enalapril. It may result in decreased formation of the active metabolite of clopidogrel, resulting in high platelet reactivity in the
Clopidogrel+Sinvastatin	1	Excellent	treatment. May result in increased
ASA 100 mg+Metoprolol	1	Good	blood pressure. May result in increased risk of bradycardia and possible toxicity of
Digoxin+Metoprolol	1	Good	digital glycosides. May result in hypoglycemia or hyperglycemia; decreased
Insulin NPH+ Metoprolol	1	Good	symptoms of hypoglycemia. May result in hypoglycemia or hyperglycemia; decreased
Regular Insulin+ Metoprolol	1	Good	symptoms of hypoglycemia. May result in increased
ASA 100 mg+ Propranolol	1	Good	blood pressure.
Captopril+Chlorpromazine	1	Excellent	May result in hypotension.

*Interaction may cause exacerbation of the patient's condition and/or require a change in treatment (Micromedex® Solutions, 2018).

The dose is an important factor in interactions with ASA. We only found prescriptions with a dosage of 100 mg, which in the elderly, use at this dosage is indicated as a platelet antiaggregant

(ARAUJO and MENEZES, 2012).

In this context, the study showed that the number of drug interactions is directly proportional to the number of drugs and comorbidities and showed that interaction is a highly frequent event in the elderly people treated in primary care included in the study.

The interactions observed and quantified in Table 5 indicate the prevalence of ASA interactions with antihypertensive drugs (Propranolol, enalapril, captopril and metroprolol), which according to Micromedex® Solutions (2018), this interaction is associated with a decrease in the therapeutic efficacy of antihypertensive drugs, resulting in a lack of BP control.

In the present study, we obtained a prevalence of 24 moderate drug interactions, similar to the prevalence found in the study by Garske, et al (2016), which also showed ASA (23.8%) as the most prevalent. Pinto, et al (2014), also carried out a study of drug interactions in patients treated at a basic health unit in Ribeirâo Preto/SP with 40 elderly people, and found a higher prevalence of interactions with AAS.

The results shown in Table 6 reveal the 19 drug interactions classified as major, in which ASA 100 mg associated with hydrochlorothiazide was the most recurrent (5).

Table 6- Most frequent Major drug interactions and <u>available</u> scientific evidence. <u>ESF 13, Juazeiro do Norte/CE, 2018.</u>

Major* type interactions	Prevalence (n=19)	Evidence Scientific	Clinical effects on the patient
Fluoxetine+ Propranolol	2	Good	It can result in an increased risk of toxicity with propranolol, including complete heart block.
Hydrochlorothiazide+ Ibuprofen	2	Good	It can result in reduced diuretic efficacy and possible nephrotoxicity.

Anlodipine + Simvastatin	2	Good	It can result in increased exposure to simvastatin and an increased risk of myopathy, including rhabdomyolysis.
ASA 100 mg+ Hydrochlorothiazide	5	Good	It can result in reduced diuretic efficacy and possible nephrotoxicity.
ASA 100 mg+ Furosemide	1	Good	It can result in reduced diuretic efficacy and possible nephrotoxicity.
ASA 100 mg+ Spironolactone	1	Good	It may result in reduced diuretic efficacy, hyperkalemia or possible nephrotoxicity.
Digoxin+ Spironolactone	2	Good	May result in increased exposure to digoxin.
Clopidogrel+ Omeprazole	1	Excellent	It may result in reduced plasma concentrations of the active metabolite of clopidogrel and reduced antiplatelet activity.

Captopril+Digoxin	1	Good	It may result in an increase in digoxin plasma concentrations.
Diazepam+ Phenobarbital	1	Good	It can result in additive respiratory depression.
Amitriptyline + ASA 100 mg	1	Excellent	It can result in an increased risk of bleeding.

* Interaction may be life-threatening and/or require medical intervention to minimize or avoid serious adverse effects (Micromedex® Solutions, 2018).

The serious drug interactions detected in this study, especially those between ASA and antihypertensive drugs (hydrochlorothiazide, furosemide, spironolactone), can result in serious harm to elderly patients, the most common being nephrotoxicity. This is important because in the elderly there is a decrease in renal flow and glomerular filtration; therefore, when drugs are excreted via the kidneys, an increase in their half-life can be observed, which can result in accumulation and toxicity (CUENTRO, *et al.*, 2014).

Another important interaction detected was between digoxin x captopril and digoxin x spironolactone, both of which pose a potential risk of digitalis intoxication. In addition, digoxin, a drug considered unsuitable for elderly patients according to the Brazilian consensus on MPI (2016), had significant interactions and was outside the recommended dose (<0.125mg). An analysis by Lutz, Miranda and Bertoldi (2017) found a similar result, in which 55.3% of elderly people using digoxin were on a potentially inadequate dose.

Soares, et al (2011), reported the same serious interactions that occur with drugs found in this study, in particular the interaction between Anlodipine and simvastatin (2), that when administered together, Anlodipine increases exposure to simvastatin and there is an increased risk of myopathies, including rhabdomyolysis.

The Food and Drug Administration (FDA) recommends that if concomitant use of these drugs is necessary, the dose of simvastatin should not exceed 20 mg/day.

In clinical practice and considering that the elderly have a complex pharmacotherapy, it is common for prescribed drugs to have drug interactions at some point (SILVA, SCHMIDIT and SILVA, 2012).

Pharmacotherapy in these patients is also affected, which requires special care, given the peculiarities presented in pharmacokinetic and pharmacodynamic parameters (MASCARENHAS *et al*; 2014). In this sense, it is important that the health team, in which the pharmacist must be included, knows how to ensure safe and effective pharmacotherapy, in which the recognition of potential drug interactions, whether moderate or severe, should be part of the care provided to elderly patients.

Although the control and treatment of most diseases are linked to the use of drug therapy, it is necessary to consider that in the elderly, pharmacotherapy has particularities that can somehow contribute to adverse reactions, including those characterized as iatrogenic.

Table 7 shows the pharmaceutical analysis of potentially inappropriate medications for the elderly, according to the classification of the Brazilian Consensus on PIM (2016), found in the prescriptions, which totaled 19 active ingredients that were contraindicated.

Table 7- Characterization of Potentially Inappropriate Medications for the Elderly, Regardless of Clinical Condition. ESF 13, Juazeiro do Norte/CE, 2018.

Class of Medicines		n	%
Central Nervous System and Psychotropic Drugs		11	22,00
Cardiovascular System		4	8,00
Gastrointestinal System		2	4,00
Musculoskeletal System		2	4,00
MPI in the elderly found in medical prescriptions	Rational	n	%

Digoxin 0.25 mg	The decrease in renal clearance with age increases the risk of digitalis intoxication. Furthermore, in CHF, higher doses increase the risk of toxicity and do not offer greater benefits.	3	6,00
Glibenclamide	Increased risk of severe prolonged hypoglycemia in the elderly.	9	18,00
Omeprazole	Potential for developing osteoporosis/fractures, dementia and kidney failure with prolonged use.	38	76,00
Diazepam	increase the risk of cognitive impairment, delirium, falls, fractures and automobile accidents. benzodiazepines to treat insomnia, agitation or delirium.	5	10,00

Phenobarbital	High proportion of physical dependence, tolerability in inducing sleep and risk of overdose at low doses.	2	4,00
		2	4,00
Spironolactone	Risk of hyperkalemia in patients with CHF, especially with concomitant use of NSAIDs, ACEIs or angiotensin receptor blockers.	7	14,00
Amitriptyline	Highly anticholinergic, sedative and cause orthostatic hypotension.		

Clonazepam	increase the risk of cognitive impairment, delirium, falls, fractures and automobile accidents. benzodiazepines to treat insomnia, agitation or delirium.	2	4,00
Chlorpromazine	Increased risk of stroke and mortality	2	4,00
Promethazine	Risk of sedation and anticholinergic effects. Tolerance develops when used as hypnotics.	2	4,00
Biperidene	Risk of anticholinergic toxicity	1	2,00

		2	4,00
Ibuprofen	They increase the risk of gastrointestinal bleeding and peptic ulcer in high-risk groups, including those aged > 75 years.	1	2,00
Nortriptyline	Highly anticholinergic, sedative and cause orthostatic hypotension.		
Furosemide	There are safer and more effective alternatives.	3	6,00
		1	2,00
Phenytoin	Risk of confusion, hypotension, extrapyramidal effects and falls.	1	2,00
Amiodarone	It is associated with thyroid disease, lung disorders and prolongation of the QT interval.		

The study revealed that of the drugs prescribed for the elderly recorded in the medical records, 22% were drugs that act on the central nervous system and 8% that act on the cardiovascular system, being considered inappropriate regardless of the clinical condition, with a high level of evidence and a strong degree of recommendation for non-use in the elderly.

Of the drugs used to control diabetes, we found a prevalence of Glibenclamide of 18% (n=9), similar to the consumption pattern found in the studies carried out by Lutz, Miranda and Bertoldi (2017).

In relation to dosage, the only drug that was totally inappropriate in this parameter was digoxin. According to the MPI consensus (2016), even in conditions of heart failure, this drug should not be prescribed at a dose of more than 0.125 mg/day, given the physiological changes at renal level, which could precipitate digitalis intoxication.

This drug in particular predisposes elderly patients to an increased risk of hypoglycemia and is therefore considered an MPI (OLIVERA, et al, 2016).

In a study carried out by Huffenbaecher, Varalho and Mastroianni (2012), which aimed to analyze the occurrence of inappropriate medications for the elderly in the family health strategy in the municipality of Araraquara/SP, they also found that of the 103 prescriptions evaluated, 47.6% were PIMs that acted on the central nervous system and 31.7% on the cardiovascular system, based on the Beers criteria.

The most commonly prescribed drugs that act on the central nervous system, considered to be PIMs, were: Amitriptyline (14%; n=7) and Diazepam (10%; n=5), classified respectively as tricyclic antidepressants and benzodiazepines (BZD). The same category of drugs was found in Huffenbaecher, Varalho and Mastroianni (2012).

Oliveira *et al.* (2009) found that the use of psychotropic drugs in four ESF units in Marília (SP) was around 11%. Factors that justify the high consumption of these drugs derive from the profile of chronic and continuous use of these substances by adults and the elderly and pharmacodependence (CRUZ *et al.*, 2014).

Medicines used by the elderly studied by Coelho Filho; Marcopito and Castelo (2004), in Fortaleza/CE, revealed that more than 80.0% of the drugs were considered PIMs, with long-acting benzodiazepines being the most inappropriate with the highest proportion of use in the elderly, where almost 7.0% of them were using at least one drug belonging to this group. In Aracaju/SE, Aguiar et al. (2008), carrying out a study in nursing homes, found that 28.7% of the elderly used at least one PIM, among which the most commonly used were amitriptyline (23.1%), amiodarone (20.5%) and thioridazine (15.4%).

Diazepam (10%) and Clonazepam (4%), drugs also considered to be PIMs, had the same prescription profile found in the studies by Naloto, et al (2016). As described in the medical records, these drugs were used as therapy for insomnia, are long-acting benzodiazepines and are considered PIMs, regardless of the clinical condition. They have a long half-life in the elderly, which produces prolonged sedation, psychomotor alterations, lack of coordination, increased risk of falls and fractures, the use of these drugs is contraindicated in the elderly. (OLIVEIRA, et al, 2016).

Even though BZDs are clinically prescribed to the elderly, evidence shows that with age, there are significant changes in the gabaergic complex, particularly in relation to GABA receptors, which are responsible for the increased sensitivity to BZDs. Other alternatives can be prescribed, such as buspirone, which can be prescribed in cases of anxiety, as well as having a short half-life and an anxiolytic effect without causing sedation, dependence or withdrawal syndrome (ANDRADE, SILVA FILHO and JUNQUEIRA, 2016).

Available evidence evaluating the clinical effectiveness and cost-effectiveness of BZDs in the elderly suggests a greater chance of adverse cognitive and psychomotor events, such as falls and fractures. No study has accurately assessed the safety, clinical efficacy and cost-effectiveness of BZD use in the treatment of anxiety or behavioral problems in the elderly (ALVARENGA, et al, 2015).

When we analyzed the use of antidepressants in the elderly, we found that Amitriptyline was the most prescribed 7 (14%). Araújo, et al (2012), when investigating the supply of antidepressants by medicine units in the CSFs of the headquarters and districts of the municipality of Sobral/CE, obtained a prevalence of 44.62% of dispensing Amitriptyline 25 mg.

Lopes, et al (2016), found 11 (21.5%) prescriptions for tricyclic antidepressants in elderly patients. In an investigation into the use of antidepressants by community-dwelling elderly people, tricyclic antidepressants were also the most commonly used (76.4%) and amitriptyline (34.7%) was the predominant active ingredient (VICENTE, 2015).

Tricyclic antidepressants are considered PIMs in the elderly because they cause clinically relevant adverse effects due to their anticholinergic activity and ability to induce orthostatic hypotension and stimulation of the central nervous system, thus increasing the chances of falls and fractures (OLIVEIRA, et al, 2016).

In this context, the choice of antidepressant for the elderly should be based on the type of depression, risk of suicide, other clinical disorders and costs (SILVA, et al, 2014). This issue corroborates the Brazilian MPI criteria, which justify the use of tricyclic antidepressants in the elderly in the event of severe pain and/or depression, although the risks/benefits of prescribing should be checked (OLIVEIRA, et al, 2016).

FINAL CONSIDERATIONS

The data obtained in this study was relevant in the context of public health, as it revealed important variables relating to knowledge of the pharmacoepidemiology of potentially inappropriate medicines for the elderly. From this perspective, it also points to the need to rethink professional practice in relation to clinical pharmaceutical care for geriatric patients with polypharmacy.

It is important to note that this study has some limitations. As the data was collected retrospectively, it is subject to variability in the system of prescribers recording information on the use of medicines at home, which can lead to a bias in the frequency of PIM. The lack of information on acute medication and self-medication are also factors to be considered, as no records were found in the medical records analyzed.

Even so, we believe that the proposed objectives were achieved and that some considerations were possible. We identified that effective pharmaceutical care for geriatric patients must be based above all on the way in which pharmacists carry out their clinical activities with these patients. Thinking only about dispensing and the pharmacy's administrative activities does not guarantee safe and effective pharmacotherapy. It is necessary to check the parameters of drug prescription in all its ethical and pharmacological aspects in order to provide active pharmaceutical care with a focus on appropriate pharmacotherapy and safety for these patients.

The study also showed a relative prevalence of the use of inappropriate medicines by elderly people treated at the FHS, according to the criteria established by the Brazilian Consensus on Potentially Inappropriate Medicines in the Elderly (2016). The prescribing behaviors of these PIMs showed a positive association with the use of polypharmacy and multiple pathologies.

The clinical consequences of PIM use in the elderly are important due to the risk of adverse events, drug iatrogenesis and the negative impact on the elderly's functionality. Highlighting these risks and presenting real data, as was done in this study, demonstrates that pharmaceutical interventions must be carried out in the context of multidisciplinary care to guarantee access to safe medicines that are appropriate to the specificities of the elderly's pharmacotherapy.

REFERENCES

ABREU, WC. Inadequate food consumption and interfering factors in the energy intake of elderly people enrolled in the municipal program for the elderly in Vinosa (MG). In: **Rev. Baiana de Saúde Pública**. V.32, n.2, 2014.

AGUIAR, P. M. et al. Evaluation of the Pharmacotherapy of Elderly Residents in Nursing Homes in Northeastern Brazil. In: **Latin American Journal of Pharmacy**, Buenos Aires, v. 27, n. 3, p. 454-459, 2008.

ALECRIM, J. de S.; CASTRO, J. M. de.; NETO, R. Z.; MIRANDA, G.M.; ALVES, R. N. CABRERA, G. P. B.; CHAGAS, A. F. S.; VAZ, A. G.; PEREIRA,G.C. A.; RUAS, H. Assessment of the pharmacotherapy used in residents of a Long-Stay Institution for the Elderly. In: **Rev. Kairós Gerontologia**. V. 19, n.3. p. 113-133, 2016.

ALVARENGA, J.M; LOYOLA FILHO, A.I.de; GIACOMIN, K.C. Use of benzodiazepines among the elderly: the relief of "throwing water on the fire", not thinking and sleeping. In: **Rev. Bras. Geriatr. Gerontol.**, Rio de Janeiro, 2015; 18(2):249-258.

ALVIM, M.M.; SILVA, L.A.; LEITE, I.C.; SILVÉRIO, M.S. Adverse events due to potential drug interactions in an intensive care unit of a teaching hospital.In: **Rev. Bras Ter Intensiva**, v. 27, n. 4, p. 353-359, 2015.

ANDRADE, K. V. F. de.; SILVA FILHO, C. da.; JUNQUEIRA, L. L. Prescribing potentially inappropriate medication for the elderly: a cross-sectional study in a psychiatric institution. In: **J. Bras. Psiquiatr**.V.62, n.2, 2016.

ANDRADE, K.V.F, de; SILVA FILHO, C, da; JUNQUEIRA, L.L. Prescription of potentially inappropriate medication for the elderly: a cross-sectional study in a psychiatric institution.In: **J. Bras. Psiquiatr**. 2016; 62 (2):149-54.

ARAUJO, B.G; MENEZES, A.C. Dosing of ASA as a platelet anti-aggregant. In: **SOUZA, P.M, ARAUJO, B.G, SILVA L.P (org.). Farmacologia clínica: textos informativos**. Brasília (DF): Universidade de Brasilia; 2012. p. 88-90.

BALDONI,A. de O; DEWULF, N. de. L. S; SANTOS, V dos. ; REIS, T. M. dos; AYRES, L. R; PEREIRA, L. R. L. Difficulties of access to pharmaceutical services by the elderly. In: **Rev. Cienc. Farm. Básica Apl**. v. 35, n. 4, 2014.

BECERRA,R. G. C; RÍOSA, E. V; RODRIGUEZA, L. G; DAZAA, E. R. V; GONZÁLERA, L. M. Estado de salud en el adulto mayor en atención primaria a partir de una valoración geriátrica integral. In: **Aten Primaria**. V. 47, n. 6, 2015.

BRAZIL. Law No. 8080/90, of September 19, 1990. Brasília: DF. 1990. Available at https://www.planalto.gov.br/ccivil_03/LEIS/L8080.htm.

BRAZIL. MINISTRY OF HEALTH. **Statute of the elderly law n°: 57, of September 23, 2003** . Brasília: Ministry of Health, 2013.

BRAZIL. MINISTRY OF HEALTH. **Strategies for the care of people with chronic diseases.** Brasilia: Ministry of Health, 2014.

BRAZIL. MINISTRY OF HEALTH. **National basic care policy. Brasilia: Ministry of Health**, 2012.

BRAZIL. MINISTRY OF HEALTH. **National health promotion policy.** Brasilia: Ministry of Health, 2010.

BRAZIL. MINISTRY OF HEALTH. **National list of essential medicines - rename 2017.** Brasilia: Ministry of Health, 2017.

Brazil. Ordinance No. 2.528, of October 19, 2006. **Approves the national health policy for the elderly**. Official Gazette of the Union, October 19, 2006.

Brazil. Ordinance No. 3.916, of October 30, 1998. **Provides for the National Medicines Policy**. Official Gazette of the Union, November 10, 1998.

Brazil. Resolution no. 338, of MAY 6, 2004. **Disposes of the National Pharmaceutical Assistance Policy**, 2004. Official Gazette of the Union, May 6, 2004.

BRAZIL. BRAZILIAN SOCIETY OF CARDIOLOGY, 2010. In: **Arq Bras Cardiol**, 2010; 95(1 supl.1): 1-51.

BUENO, C.S; OLIVEIRA, K. R. de. Potentially inappropriate medicines for the elderly: inclusion in the Municipal List of Essential Medicines of Ijuí-RS. In: **Rev. Contexto e Saúde**. v.10, n. 20, 2011.

CASAS-VÁSQUEZ P; ORTIZ-SAAVEDRA P; PENNY-MONTENEGRO. Strategies to optimize pharmacological management in older adults. **Rev. Peru Med Exp Salud Publica**. V.33, 2016.

CASCAES, E. A; FALCHETTI, M. L; GALATO, D. Profile of self-medication in elderly people participating in senior citizen groups in a city in southern Brazil. In: **Arquivos Catarinenses de Medicina, Florianópolis**, V. 37, n. 1, p. 63-69, 2008.

CASSONI, T. C. J; CORONA L. P; ROMANO, L. N. S; SECOLI, S. R; DUARTE Y. A. O; LEBRÄO M. L; Use of potentially inappropriate medication by the elderly in the Municipality of Sao Paulo, Brazil: SABE Study. In: **Cad. Saude Publica**. V.30, 2014.

CHAIMOWICZ, F. **Health of the elderly**. Belo Horizonte: Nescon/UFMG, Coopmed. 2014.

CHEHUEN NETO, J. A. et al. Use of medication by the elderly in Juiz de Fora: a look at polypharmacy. In: **HU Revista**, Juiz de Fora, v. 37, n. 3, p. 305-313, jul./set. 2012.

COBASA, P.C.R; DUQUEA, N. R; HERNANDEZ,M. G; GARCIAC, J; AGUSTID, A, X. V; FORMIGAE, F; SOTOF, A. L; TORRESG, O. H; SAN-JOSE, A. Características del uso inadecuado de medicamentos en pacientes pluripatológicos de edad avanzada. In: **Gac Sanit**. n. 31, n. 4, 2017.

CODAGNONE NETO, V; GARCIA, V.P; SANTA HELENA, E.T. Possible pharmacological interactions in hypertensive and/ or diabetic elderly in family health units at Blumenau (SC). In: **Braz J Pharm Sci**. 2010; 46: 795-804.

COELHO FILHO, J. M; MARCOPITO, L. F; CASTELO, A. Profile of medication use by the elderly in an urban area in the Northeast of Brazil. In: **Rev. Saúde Pública** [online]. 2004, vol.38, n.4, pp.557-564.

CONCEIÇÃO, A. P. de J; SARRAF, E. M; PINHEIRO, I. de M; Postural instability in the elderly during hospitalization - literature review. In: **Rev. Pesq. Em. fisioterapia. V.6. n.4, 2016.**

CORREA, L.M; RODRIGUES, C.; MACEDO, L.C. Pharmacotherapeutic evaluation in patients of a geriatric institution in the central-western region of Paraná, Brazil. In: **Rev. Saúde e Biol.**; v.11, n.1, p.22-30, jan/abr., 2016. Available   at:< http://revista.grupointegrado.br/revista/index.php/sabios2/article/view/1816>. Accessed on: June 28, 2017.

CRUZ, H.L; CRUZ, M.F.K; ANDRADE, R.A; BODEVAN, E.C; ARAÚJO, L.U; SANTOS, D.F. Caracterizaçao do uso de medicamentos entre idosos de uma unidade do Programa Saúde da Família.In: **Cad. Saúde Pública**. 2014;24(7):1545-55.

CUENTRO, V. da S; ANDRADE, M. A. de; GERLACK, L. F; BÓS, A. J. G; SILVA, M. V. S. da; OLIVEIRA, A. F. de; Drug prescriptions of patients treated at the geriatric outpatient clinic of a university hospital: a descriptive cross-sectional study. In: **Rev. Ciência & Saúde Coletiva**, V. 19, 2014.

DAL PIZZOL. Medication use among elderly people living in urban and rural areas of a municipality in southern Brazil: a population-based study. In: **Cadernos de Saúde Pública**. v. 28, n. 1, p. 104-114, 2012.

DANTAS, M.S. Use of polypharmacy among the elderly and the contribution of pharmaceutical care. In: **Rev. Especialize On-line IPOG - Goiânia**. Vol. 1, n.11, 2016.

DINIZ, J.A.; MONTAGNA, E.; CARVALHO, P.M.de. M. Inappropriate medicines for the elderly: an analysis from the perspective of the stopp criteria in the municipal list of essential medicines of a municipality in the interior of ceará. In: **Rev. Infarma de Cien. Farmacêuticas**. V.29, 2017. Available at:< http://dx.doi.org/10.14450/2318-9312.v29.esup1.a2017.pp1-286 1017>.

DOMÍNGUEZ TORRES, R; ESPINOSA, A. H; GONZALEZ, L. M. O; RODRIGUEZ, M. J. S. Polypharmacy in old age. Some considerations. **Revista Electrónica Dr. Zoilo E. Marinello Vidaurreta**, v. 38, n. 5, 2015.

ESTEVEA, I. C; MARSAL-MORAB, J. R; ORTEGA, G; SANTIAGOC, L. G; GODOYD, M. S; MURILLO, E. R; GATIUSB, J.R. Análisis poblacional de la prescripción potencialmente inadecuada en ancianos según criterios STOPP/START (estudio STARTREC). In: **Aten Primaria**. V. 49, n. 3. 2017.

FARAONI, A.S; SOUZA, C.A.S; BRITO, G. de. C, et al. Possible drug interactions among users of a basic health unit (ubs) in the municipality of sao cristóvao - SE. In: **Rev.Saúde.Com**, 2015; 11(1): 10-19.

FARIA, A. I; OBRELI-NETO, P. R; GUIDONI C. M; BALDONI, A. de O; Analysis of

Potentially Inappropriate Medicines for the Elderly contained in the Municipal List of Essential Medicines (REMUME) of Divinópolis-MG. In: **Journal of Applied Pharmaceutical Sciences** - JAPHAC. v. 2, 2015.

FASTBOM, J; JOHNELL, K. National indicators for quality of drug therapy in older persons: the Swedish experience from the first 10 years. In: **Drugs Aging**. V. 32, n. 3, 2015.

FERREIA, L. P; REZENDE, E. L. V; CORDEIRO, F. S. C; FERNANDES, F. S; MOTA, P. G. da.; VALADÄO, A.F. potentially inappropriate medicines for the elderly in the municipal list of essential medicines of Ipatinga, Minas Gerais. In:**Rev. UNINGÁ Review**. v.26,n.3, 2016.

FLORES L.M, MENGUE S.S. Uso de medicamentos por idosos em região do sul do Brasil. In: **Rev. Saúde Pública** 2005.

GALATO, D; SILVA, E.S.D; TIBURCIO, L.D.S. Study of medication use in elderly residents in a city in the south of Santa Catarina (Brazil): a look at polymedication. In: **Ciênc. saúde coletiva.** 2010.

GARCIA, M. L. N; VÁZQUEZ, M. E. S; DEMUTH, F. J. J; MANSO, G. Beers criteria versus STOPP in older, polymedicated and community-dwelling patients. In: **Farm Hosp**. V. 40, n.3,2016.

GARSKE, C. C. D; BRIXNER, B; FREITAS, A. P; SCHNEIDER, A. P. H; Evaluation of potential drug interactions in prescriptions of intensive care unit patients. In: **Rev. Saúde e Pesquisa**, v. 9, n. 3, p. 483-490, 2016.

GARSKE, C.C.D; BRIXNER, B; FREITAS, A.P; SCHNEIDER, A.P.H. Evaluation of potential drug interactions in prescriptions of intensive care unit patients. In: **Rev. Saúde e Pesquisa**, v. 9, n. 3, p. 483-490, Sep./Dec. 2016.

GIL, A.C. **Métodos e Técnicas de Pesquisa Social**. Sao Paulo: Atlas, 2008.

GOODMAN, A. As Bases Farmacológicas da Terapêutica. 11. ed. Rio de Janeiro: McGraw-Hill, 2006.

GOMES, J. L. de.; COSTA,M.da.C; MELO, R. J. P; LUCENA, A.; SANTOS, M. A. M dos.; GUIMARÄES,F.J. de. Sá. P. Effectiveness of a combined exercise program on anthropometric variables, body composition and neuromotor tests in elderly women. In: **Rev. Brasileira de Prescriçâo e Fisiologia do Exercício**. V. 11. n.67. p.469-477,2017.

GONTIJO, M.D.F; RIBEIRO, A.Q; KLEIN, C.H; ROZENFELD, S; ACURCIO, F.A. Use of antihypertensives and antidiabetics by the elderly: a survey in Belo Horizonte, Minas Gerais, Brazil. In: **Cad Saude Publica**. 2012;28 (7):1337-46.

GORARD, D. A. Escalating polypharmacy. QJM: monthly journal of the Association of Physicians, Oxford, v. 99, n. 11, p. 797-800, 2006.

GORZONI, M.L; FABBRI, R.M; PIRES, S.L. Medicamentos Potencialmente Inapropriados para Idodos.In: **Rev. Assoc. Med. Bras.** 2012, vol.58, n. 4, p. 442-446. Available at:< http://www.scielo.br/pdf/ramb/v58n4/v58n4a14.pdf>. Accessed on: March 22, 2016.

GOULART, L. S; CARVALHO, A. C; LIMA, J. C; PEDROSA, J. M , LEMOS, P. de L; OLIVEIRA, R. B. Consumo de medicamentos por um idosos de um unidade basi ca de saúde de rondonópolis/MT. In: **Estud. interdiscipl. envelhec.** V. 19, n. 1, p. 79-94, 2014.

GOULART, LS; CARVALHO, A.C; LIMA, J.C; PEDROSA, J.M; LEMOS, P.L; OLIVEIRA, R.B. Consumo de medicamentos por idosos de uma unidade básica de saúde de Rondonópolis/MT. In: **Estud. Interdiscip. Envelhec.** 2014;19(1):79-94.

GUIMARAES, P.L; MOURA, C.S. Factors associated with the use of inappropriate high-risk medications in hospitalized elderly patients. In: **Rev. Bras. Farm. Hosp. Ser. Saúde**. Sao Paulo, v.3, n.4. oct./dec. 2012.   p.   15-19.   Available   at:< http://www.sbrafh.org.br/rbfhss/public/artigos/2012030418BR.pdf>. Accessed on: March 18, 2016.

HILARIO, I.D.; SIMONETTI, E.; RIGO, M. P. M; CASTRO, L.C. de.; KAUFFMANN, C. Analysis of pharmacotherapy in an elderly care center in the taquari valley - RS. In: **Caderno pedagógico**, Lajeado, v. 12, n. 3, p. 101-116, 2015.

HIPÓLITO P, ROCHA BS, OLIVEIRA, FJAQ. Profile of users prescribed omeprazole in a Basic Health Unit in Southern Brazil: considerations on its rational use.In: **Rev. Bras. Med. Fam. Comunidade.** 2016;11(38):1-10. http://dx.doi.org/10.5712/rbmfc11(38)1153.

HUFFENBAECHER, P.; VARALLO, F. R.; MASTROIANNI, P. C. Inadequate medication for the elderly in the family health strategy. In: **Rev. Ciência em Extensäo**, v. 8, n. 3, p. 56-67, 2012.

BRAZILIAN INSTITUTE OF GEOGRAPHY AND STATISTICS (IBGE). Demographic Census, 2010.

BRAZILIAN INSTITUTE OF GEOGRAPHY AND STATISTICS (IBGE). National health survey 2013, perception of health status, lifestyles and chronic diseases. ftp://ftp.ibge.gov.br/PNS/2013/pns2013.pdf.

JARDIM, R. BARRETO, S.M; GIATTI, L. Reliability of information obtained from secondary informants in health surveys. In: **Cad. Saúde Pública,** 2010; 26:1537-48.

LIMA, A.P.V; NETO, FILHO, M.A. Long-term effects of proton pump inhibitors. In: **Braz. J Surg Clin Res.** 2013:5(3):45-9.

LIMA, T. A.M. de.; FAZAN, E.R.; PEREIRA, L.L.V.; GODOY, M.F.de. Pharmacotherapeutic follow-up in the elderly. In: **Arq. Ciênc. Saúde.** V. 23, n.1, 2016.

LINJAKUMPU T; HARTIKAINEN S; KLAUKKA T; VEIJOLA J; KIVELÄ S.L; ISOAHO R. Use of medications and polypharmacy are increasing among the elderly. In: **J Clin Epidemiol,** 2002.

LINO A.S. **Comparison of lipid and protein profile between sedentary adults and active elderly in a selected population of the city of Patos -PB**. Informativo Técnico do Semiárido, 2015.

LOPES, L.M; FIGUEIREDO, T.P.de; COSTA, S.C; REIS, A.M.M. Utilizaçao de medicamentos potencialmente inapropriadas por idosos em domicílio.In: **Ciência & Saúde Coletiva,** 21(11):3429- 3438, 2016.

LOYOLA FILHO, A.I; UCHOA, E; LIMA-COSTA, M.F. Population-based study on medication consumption among the elderly: Bambuí Project. In: **Cad Saúde Pública,** 2005.

LUTZ, B. H; MIRANDA,V.I. A; BERTOLDI, A. D. Inadequate use of medication among the elderly in Pelotas, RS. In: **Rev. Saude Publica.** 2017.

MALACHIAS, M.V.B; SOUZA, W.K.S.B; PLAVNIK, F.L; RODRIGUES, C.I.S; BRANDÄO, A,A; NEVES, M.F.T, et al. 7ª Diretriz Brasileira de Hipertensao Arterial. In: **Arq. Bras Cardiol,** 2016; 107(3Supl.3):1-83.

MALAQUIAS, B. S. S; BUSO, A. L. Z; SILVANO, C. M; NARDELLI, G. G; MARTINS G. T; SANTOS, A. S; Evaluation of drug prescriptions to the elderly in a geriatric outpatient clinic.In: **Rev. Medicina (Ribeiräo Preto. Online)** V. 49, 2016.

MALTA, D.C; BERNAL, R.T.I; LIMA, M.G; ARAÚJO, S.S.C; SILVA, M.M.A; FREITAS, M.I.F, et al. Chronic non-communicable diseases and the use of health services: an analysis of the National Health Survey in Brazil. In: **Rev. Saude Publica.** 2017;51 Supl 1:4s.

MANSO,M. E. G.; BIFFI, E.C. A.; GERARDI, T. J. Inadequate prescribing of medication to elderly people with chronic diseases in a health plan in the municipality of Sao Paulo, Brazil.In: **Rev. Bras. Geriatr. Gerontol.,** v. 18, n. 1,2015.

MARIN, M. J. S; CECÍLIO, L. C. de O; PEREZ, A. E. W. U. F; SANTELLA, F; SILVA, C. B. A; FILHO, J. R. G; ROCETI, L. C; Characterization of medication use among the elderly in a Family Health Program unit. In: REV. **Cad Saúde Pública,**V.24, 2008.

MASCARENHAS, G. D.de. M; SILVA, K.O; SILVA, P.Z. da.; FARIA, L. A.de.; REIS, L.A. dos.; NOVAIS, M.I. Adequacy of medication used by elderly participants in a community group, according to the Beers criteria. In: **Rev.Saúde.Com** . v.14, n. 3., 201 4.

MEDEIROS, P. Diagnosis and control of polypharmacy in the elderly. In: **Rev. de Saúde Pública** v. 41, n. 6, p. 1049-1053, 2007.

MICROMEDEX® Solutions [Internet]. Accessed: March 14, 2018. Available at: http://wwwmicromedexsolutionscom.ez127.periodicos.capes.gov.br/micromedex2/librarian.

MOTA, M. S. P. Diagnosis of an elderly population. In: **Rev. Estudos Interdisciplinares sobre o Envelhecimento.** v. 15, n. 2, p. 255-264, 2010.

MUNIZ, E. C. S; GOULART, F. C; LAZARINI, C. A; MARIN, M. J. S. Analysis of the use of medication by elderly users of supplementary health insurance. In: **Rev. Bras. Geriatr. Gerontol.,** V. 20, n. 3. 2017.

MUÑOZ, R.L. de. S; IBIAPINA, G.R; GADELHA, C.S; MARAJA, J.L.S. Inappropriate geriatric prescriptions and polypharmacotherapy in medical wards of a Teaching Hospital. In: **Rev. Bras. Geriatr. Gerontol**; Rio de Janeiro, 2012; v.15, n. 2. p. 315-323. Available at:< http://www.scielo.br/pdf/rbgg/v15n2/14.pdf>. Accessed on: March 14, 2016.

NAKATA, K. C. de F; SILVA, L. M. V. Avaliação da Acessibilidade à Assistência Farmacéutica Básica no Município de Várzea Grande (Mato Grosso). In: **Rev Ciênc Farm**

Básica Apl. v.35, n: 3, 2014.

NALOTO, D.C.C; LOPES, F.C; BARBERATO-FILHO, S, et al. Prescription of benzodiazepines for adults and the elderly in a mental health outpatient clinic. In: **Ciência & Saúde Coletiva**, 21(4):1267-1276, 2016.

NASCIMENTO JUNIOR, J. M. do; ALEXANDRE, R. F; COSTA, L. H; SANTOS, R. S; LUPATINI, E. de O; DOMINGUES, P. H. F; BIELA, C. de A. . RENAME's progress and prospects after the new legal frameworks: the challenge of contributing to a single, comprehensive SUS. In: **Rev. Eletrônica Gestäo & Saúde**. v. 6,2015.

O'MAHONY D; O'SULLIVAN, D; BYRNE, S; O'CONNOR, M.N; RYAN, C, G. P. STOPP/START criteria for potentially inappropriate prescribing in older people: version 2. In: **Ageing Ageing**, v. 44, n. 2, 2015.

OLIVEIRA, C.A.P; MARIN, M.J.S; MARCHIOLI, M; PIZOLETTO, B.H.M; SANTOS, R.V. Caracterizaçao dos medicamentos prescritos aos idosos na estratégia saúde da família. In: **Cad. Saude Publica**. 2009;25(5):1007-16.

OLIVEIRA, M.A; LUIZA, V.L; TAVARES, N.U.L; MENGUE, S.S; ARRAIS, P.S.D; FARIAS, M.R, *et al*. Access to medicines for chronic diseases in Brazil: a multidimensional approach. In: **Rev. Saude Publica**. 2016;50 (supl 2):6s.

OLIVEIRA, M.G; AMORIM, W.W; OLIVEIRA, C.R.B; COQUEIRO, H.L; GUSMÄO, L.C; PASSOS, L.C. Consenso brasileiro de medicamentos potencialmente inapropriados para idosos. In: **Geriatrics, Gerontology and Aging**. V. 10, n. 4, p. 1-14, 2016. Available at: < http://www.ggaging.com/details/397/pt-BR/brazilian-consensus-of-potentially-inappropriate-medication-for-elderly-people>.

OLIVEIRA, M.G; AMORIM, W.W; RODRIGUES, V.A; PASSOS, L.C. Access to potentially inappropriate medicines in the elderly in Brazil. In: **Rev APS**. 2011;14(3):258-65.

OLIVEIRA, R. E. M. de; NASCIMENTO. M. M. G. do.; PEREIRA, M. L. Use of medication by the elderly in a primary health care unit. In: **Rev. Bras. Farm. Hosp. Serv. Saúde Säo Paulo**. v.7 n.3, p. 30-34, 2016.

WORLD HEALTH ORGANIZATION. World report on ageing and health 2015. Available at: < http://sbgg.org.br/wp-content/uploads/2015/10/OMS-ENVELHECIMENTO- 2015-port.pdf.

PARENTE, A.M.E. G. **Estado nutricional dos idosos no Centro de Saúde Santa Maria de Bragança**. Dissertation (Master's Degree in Community Nursing) - School of Health. Instituto Politécnico de Bragança, Bragança, 2016; 210p.

PERIQUITO, C.M.de. N; SILVA, P.C; OLIVEIRA, P; CARNEIRO, C; FERNANDES, A.I; COSTA, F.A, da. Review of Medication in Institutionalized Elderly: Application of the STOPP and START Criteria.In: **Rev. Port. Farmacoter**. 2014, vol. 6, p. 211-220. Available at:< http://www.usoresponsaveldomedicamento.com/documents/files/artigo_3.pdf>. Accessed on: March 10, 2016.

PINTO, N.B.F; VIEIRA, L.B; PEREIRA, F.M.V. et al.; Drug interactions in prescriptions of elderly hypertensive patients: prevalence and clinical significance. In: **Rev. enferm UERJ**, Rio de Janeiro, 2014 Nov/Dec; 22(6):735-41.

POULTER,N.R; PRABHAKARAN,D; CAULFIELD, M. Hypertension. In: **Lancet**. 2015;386(9995):801-12.

RAMOS L.R; TAVARES, N.U.L; BERTOLDI, A.D; FARIAS, M.R; OLIVEIRA, M.A; LUIZA, V.L, et al. Polypharmacy and polymorbidity in the elderly in Brazil: a public health challenge. In: **Rev. Saude Publica**. 2016;50(supl 2):9s.

RODRIGUES, M. C. S; OLIVEIRA, C. de. Drug interactions and adverse drug reactions in polypharmacy in the elderly: an integrative review. In: **Rev. Latino-Am. Enfermagem**. 2016.

SALECH, F; PALMA, D; GARRIDO, P. Epidemiología del uso de medicamentos en el adulto mayor. In: **Rev. Med. Clin. Condes**, V.27, n.5, 2016.

SALES, A.S.; SALES, M.G.S.; CASOTTI, C.A. Pharmacotherapeutic profile and factors associated with polypharmacy among the elderly in Aiquara, Bahia, in 2014. In: **Epidemiol. Serv. Saude**. V.26, n.1,. 2017.

SANCHE, J. F; GARDENGI, G. Ageing and its relationship with nutritional status and physical exercise. Available at:< http://www.ceafi.com.br/biblioteca/o-envelhecimento-e-sua-relationship-with-nutritional-status-and-physical-exercise>.

SANTOS, A.M.dos; CARNEIRO, L.S; CHAUD, L.C.S; URIAS, G.M.P.C; BRUM, H.C.C. Study of the pharmacotherapeutic profile of elderly patients with type II diabetes. In: **Rev. Ciên.**

Saúde v. 1, n. 3, 2016.
SANTOS, G. S; CUNHA, I. C. K. O. Factores asociados al consumo de medicamentos entre ancianos de una unidad básica de salud. In: **REFACS (online)**. V. 5, n.2. 2017.
SANTOS, T. R. A; LIMA, D. M; NAKATANI, A. Y. K; PEREIRA, L. V; LEAL, G. S AMARAL, R. G. Consumption of medicines by the elderly, Goiânia, Brazil. In: **Rev. Saúde Pública**, V. 47, n. 1, 2013.
SCALA, L.C; MAGALHÂES, L.B; MACHADO, A. Epidemiology of systemic arterial hypertension. In: **MOREIRA, S.M; PAOLA, A.V; Brazilian Society of Cardiology. Textbook of the Brazilian Society of Cardiology**. 2ª . ed. Sao Pauilo: Manole; 2015. p. 780-5.
SILVA, A. L. da; RIBEIRO, A. Q.; KLEIN, C. H; ACURCIO, F. de A; Medication use by elderly Brazilians, according to age group: a postal survey. In: **Cad. Saúde Pública**, V. 28, 2012.
SILVA, J.R; VARGEM, D.da. S; SOUSA, M.C.de; PINTO, I.B. O Consumo de Amitriptilina e Nortriptilina no Hospital Espírita Psiquiátrico de Anápolis. In: **Ensaios Cienc., Cienc. Biol. Agrar. Saúde**, v. 18, n. 1, p. 3-8, 2014.
SILVA, L.D.; SANTOS, M.M. Drug Interactions in the Intensive Care Unit: A Review that Underpins Nursing Care. In: **Rev. de Enfermagem**. Rio de Janeiro, v. 19, n. 1, p. 139 - 139. 2011.
SILVA, R. M; OLIVEIRA, D. W. D. de; BISCARO, P. C. B; ORTI, N. P; PINTO, A. C. S; JORGE, M. L. R; In: Inquérito **epidemiológico em populagá idosa (parte II): saúde bucal, ansiedade, depressáo, estresse e uso de medicamentos. Sci Med**. V.26, 2016.
SILVA, R; SCHMIDT, O.F; SILVA, S. Polypharmacy in geriatrics. In: **Rev AMRIGS**. 2012;56(2):164-74.
SOARES, M.A; FERNANDEZ-LLIMOS, F; CABRITA, J ; MORAIS, J. Tools to evaluate potentially inappropriate prescription in the elderly: a systematic review. In: **Acta Med Port**. 2011; 24: 775-84.
SONNICHSEN, A; TRAMPISCH, U.S; RIECKERT,A; PICCOLIORI, G; VOGELE, A; FLAMM, M. Polypharmacy in chronic diseases-Reduction of Inappropriate Medication and Adverse drug events in older populations by electronic Decision Support (PRIMA-eDS): study protocol for a randomized controlled trial. In: **Trials**.v. 1, n.1, 2016.
SOUZA, I.K.F; SILVA, A.L; ARAÚJO, JÚNIOR, A; SANTOS, F.C.B; MENDONCA, B.P.C.K. Qualitative analysis of anatomopathological changes in the gastric mucosa resulting from prolonged therapy with proton pump inhibitors: experimental studies x clinical studies.In: **Arq Bras Cir Dig**. 2013;26(4):328-34.
TAVARES, E.L; SANTOS, D.M. dos; FERREIRA, A.A; MENEZES, M.F. G.de. Nutritional assessment of the elderly: current challenges. In: Rev. **Brasileira de Geriatria e Gerontologia**, V.18, n. 3, 2015.
TAVARES, M. C. S de; LIMA, C. M. V. Dificuldades do idoso e familiares na medicagao domiciliar.In: **Rev. INTERFACES**, v.4, n. 12, 2017.
TAVARES, N.U.L; LUIZA, V.L; OLIVEIRA, M.A; COSTA, K.S; MENGUE, S.S; ARRAIS, P.S.D; et al. Free access to medicines for the treatment of chronic diseases in Brazil. In: **Rev. Saude Publica**. 2016;50(supl 2):7s.
TERASSI, M; RISSARDO, L; PEIXOTO, J; SALCI, M; CARREIRA, L. Prevalence of drug use in institutionalized elderly: a descriptive study Online Brazilian Journal of Nursing [serial on the Internet]. 2012 April 18; [Cited 2012 May 11]; 11(1).
TEIXEIRA, J.C.F.C. **Geriatric pharmacokinetics**. Master's thesis. University Fernando Pessoa. 2015.
VARALLO, F.R; COSTA, M.A; MASTROIANNI, P.C. Potential drug interactions responsible for hospital interactions. In: **Rev. Ciênc. Farm. Básica Apl**. 2013; 34(1):79-85.
VÁSQUEZ, P. C; SAAVEDRA, P. O; MONTENEGRO, E. P; estrategias para optimizar el manejo farmacológico en el adulto mayor. In: **Rev. Peru Med Exp Salud Publica**. V.33, 2016.
VICENTE, A.R.T. Antidepressant consumption among the elderly: Evidence from the Bambuí project / Adriano Roberto Tarifa Vicente. - Belo Horizonte, 2015.
VRDOLJAK, D BOROVAC, J.A.. Medication in the elderly-considerations and therapy prescription guidelines. In: **Acta Med Acad**. V. 44, n.2, p. 159-68. 2015.

APPENDIX

APPENDIX A - STANDARDIZED FORMS

PATIENT PROFILE
Date of birth:___________ //
Age:
Gender: [ ] Male [ ] Female

MEDICAL DIAGNOSIS HEALTH PROBLEMS [Record patient's health problems]

PATIENT'S HEALTH PROBLEMS	Current Clinical Status (TT= TREATED; NTT= NOT TREATED)
1.	
2.	
3.	
4.	
5.	
6.	
7.	

PHARMACEUTICAL EVALUATION I - CURRENT PHARMACOTHERAPY

Active ingredient/Concentration/Pharmaceutical form	Prescribed dosage	Origin of Prescription	Indication Clinic

PHARMACEUTICAL EVALUATION II

PROBLEMS RELATED TO PHARMACOTHERAPY

problems involving selection and prescription

[ ] **Prescribing inappropriate or contraindicated medication**
[ ] **Prescription drug with no defined clinical indication**
[ ] **Prescribe in subdose**
[ ] **Prescribe in overdose**
[ ] **Inadequate frequency or timing of prescribed administration**
[ ] **Duration of treatment prescribed inadequate**
[ ] **Drug-drug interaction**
[ ] **Omission of prescribed medication**
[ ] **Duplicate therapy between prescribers**

PHARMACEUTICAL EVALUATION III

CRITERIA OF THE BRAZILIAN CONSENSUS ON INAPPROPRIATE MEDICATION IN THE ELDERLY (2016)	
.1 CARDIOVASCULAR SYSTEM	
.2 CENTRAL NERVOUS SYSTEM	
.3 GASTROINTESTINAL SYSTEM	
.4 RESPIRATORY SYSTEM	
.5 MUSCULOSKELETAL SYSTEM	
.6 URINARY SYSTEM	
.7 ENDOCRINE SYSTEM	
.8 DRUGS WITH ADVERSE EFFECTS IN PEOPLE AT HIGH RISK OF FALLING	

.9 ANALGESIC DRUGS	
10 DUPLICATE DRUGS (SAME PHARMACOLOGICAL CLASS)	

Source: Brazil. Ministry of Health. Capacitando para implantando dos servaos de clínica farmacéutica, 2017.

ANNEX B- DRUGS THAT SHOULD BE AVOIDED IN THE ELDERLY REGARDLESS OF CLINICAL CONDITION, ACCORDING TO THE BRAZILIAN MPI CONSENSUS
(2016)

Central Nervous System		
Pharmacological Class	**Medicines**	**Justification Inadequacy**
Antiparkinsonian	Biperidene	Risk of anticholinergic toxicity
	Triexifenidil	
1st generation antihistamines	Bronfeniramine	Risk of sedation and anticholinergic effects (confusion, dry mouth, constipation, among others). Tolerance develops when used as a hypnotic.
	Carbinoxamine	
	Ciproeptadine	

	Clemastine	
	Chlorpheniramine	
	Dexchlorpheniramine	
	Diphenhydramine	
	Dimenhydrinate	
	Doxylamine	
	Hydroxyzine	
	Meclizine	
	Promethazine	
	Triprolidine	

First-generation antipsychotics	Chlorpromazine	Increased risk of stroke and mortality.
	Flufenazine	
	Haloperidol	
	Levomepromazine	
	Penfluridol	
	Periciazine	
	Pimozide	
	Pipothiazide	
	Sulpiride	
	Thioridazine	

	Trufluoperazine	
	Zuclopentixol	
Barbiturates	Phenobarbital	High propensity of physical dependence, tolerance in sleep induction and risk of overdose at low doses
	Thiopental	
Benzodiazepines	Alprazolam	Increases the risk of cognitive impairment, delirium, falls, fractures and automobile accidents. Avoid for treatment of insomnia, agitation or delirium.
	Bromazepam	
	Clobazam	
	Clonazepam	
	Chlordiazepoxide	
	Cloxazolam	

	Diazepam	
	Estazolam	
	Flunitrazepam	
	Flurazepam	
	Lorazepam	
	Midazolam	
	Nitrazepam	
Non-benzodiazepine hypnotics	Zolpidem (>90) days	Similar effects to benzodiazepines
Tertiary tricyclic antidepressants	Amitriptyline	Anticholinergic, sedative effects and causes orthostatic hypotension
	Imipramine	

	Nortriptyline	
	Clomipramine	
	Maprotiline	

	Cardiovascular System	
Pharmacological Class	**Medicines**	**Justification Inadequacy**
Alpha-1 blockers to treat hypertension	Doxazosin	High risk of orthostatic hypotension
	Prazosin	
	Terazosin	
Centrally acting alpha agonists	Clonidine	Risk of adverse effects on the CNS.
	Methyldopa	

	Reserpine > 0.1 mg/day	
Antiarrhythmics la, Ic, III	Amiodarone	Bradycardia, orthostatic hypotension
	Propafenone	
	Quinidine	
	Sotalol	
NSAIDS	Aspirin > 150 mg/day	Increases the risk of digestive bleeding
Glycosides	Digoxin > 0.125 mg/day	Digit poisoning , due to decreased renal clearance
Alkaline diuretics for ankle edema, in the absence of clinical signs of heart failure	Bumetanide	No evidence of effectiveness
	Furosemide	
	Pyrethanide	

Alkyl diuretics as 1st line therapy for hypertension	Bumetanide	
	Furosemide	Safer and more effective alternatives
	Pyrethanide	
Calcium channel blocker	Nifedipine, extended-release capsule	Potential for hypotension. Risk of myocardial ischemia
Potassium-sparing diuretic	Spironolacotone > 25 mg/day (patients with heart failure or CrCl < 30 mL/min)	Risk of hyperkalemia in patients with heart failure
	Endocrine System	
Estrogens	With or without progesterone, avoid oral forms and transdermal patches	Evidence of carcinogenic potential (breast and endometrium)

	Androgens	Potential for heart problems and contraindicated for men with prostate cancer
Hypoglycemic	Chlorpropamide	Prolonged half-life in the elderly, can cause hypoglycemia and syndrome of inappropriate secretion of antidiuretic hormone.
Hypoglycemic	Glibenclamide	Increased risk of severe prolonged hypoglycemia in the elderly
Growth hormone	Somatoprin	Edema, arthralgia, carpal tunnel syndrome, gynecomastia and altered fasting glucose

Gastrointestinal System

Pharmacological Class	Medicines	Justification Inadequacy
Antispasmodics	Hyoscine	Highly anticholinergic. Uncertain effectiveness.

	Scopolamine	
Opioid analgesics	Loperamide	Late diagnosis can aggravate constipation with spurious diarrhea and precipitate toxic megacolon in inflammatory bowel disease and delay recovery from gastroenteritis.
	Codeine	
Dopaminergic antagonist	Metoclopramide	May cause extrapyramidal effects, including tardive dyskinesia. Increased risk for frail elderly.
Laxative	Mineral oil	Potential for aspiration and adverse effects. Safer alternatives available.
Proton pump inhibitors	Omeprazole	Potential for the development of osteoporosis/fractures, dementia and renal failure with prolonged use
	Pantoprazole	

	Lanzoprazole	
	Rabeprazole	
	Esomeprazole	
	Tenatoprazole	

Musculoskeletal system

Pharmacological Class	Medicines	Justification Inadequacy
Muscle relaxants	Carisoprodol	Increased cholinergic effect (sedation and fractures)
	Cyclobenzaprine	

	Orphenadrine	
Non-COX-selective NSAIDs	Aspirin > 325 mg/day	Increases the risk of gastrointestinal bleeding and peptic ulcer. Increases with the use of
	Diclofenac	
	Etodolaco	oral or parenteral corticosteroids, anticoagulants or antiplatelet drugs,
	Phenoprofen	
	Ibuprofen	
	Ketoprofen	
	Meloxicam	
	Naproxen	

	Piroxocam	
NSAIDS	Indomethacin and Ketorolac	They increase the risk of gastrointestinal bleeding and peptic ulcer. Indomethacin is the drug in the NSAID class that causes the most adverse effects.
Systemic corticosteroids > 3 months as monotherapy for arthritis or osteoarthritis	Betamethasone	Risk of serious adverse effects
	Budesonide	
	Deflazacorte	
	Dexamethasone	
	Fludrocortizone	
	Hydrocortizone	
	Methylprednisolone	

	Prednisolone	
	Prednisone	
Strong opioids in prolonged use as 1st line monotherapy for mild/moderate pain	Alfentanil	Does not follow the WHO analgesic scale
	Fentanyl	
	Hydromorphone	
	Methadone	
	Morphine	
	Nalbufine	
	Oxycodone	
	Pethidine	

	Remifentanil	
	Sufentanil	

Source: Brazilian Consensus on Potentially Inappropriate Medications for the Elderly (OLIVEIRA, et al, 2016).

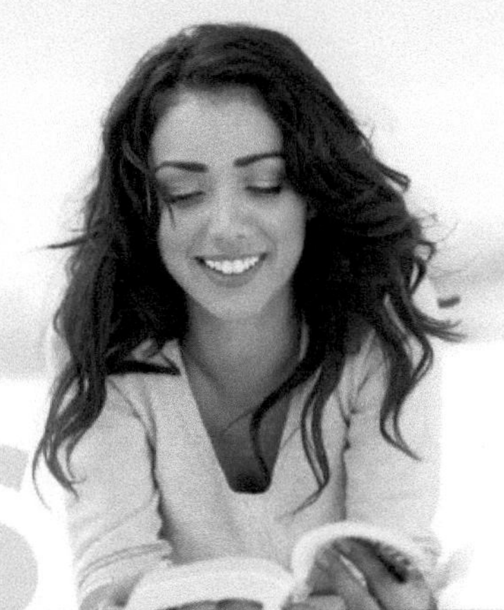

yes
I want morebooks!

Buy your books fast and straightforward online - at one of world's fastest growing online book stores! Environmentally sound due to Print-on-Demand technologies.

Buy your books online at
www.morebooks.shop

Kaufen Sie Ihre Bücher schnell und unkompliziert online – auf einer der am schnellsten wachsenden Buchhandelsplattformen weltweit! Dank Print-On-Demand umwelt- und ressourcenschonend produzi ert.

Bücher schneller online kaufen
www.morebooks.shop

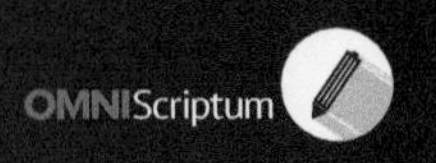

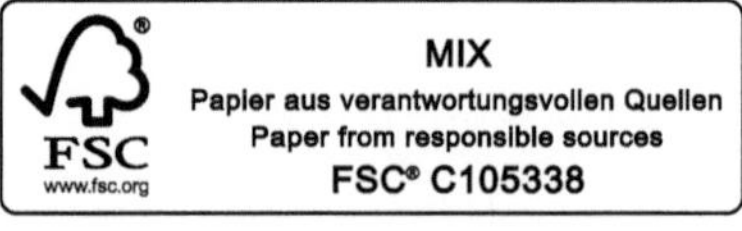

Printed by Books on Demand GmbH, Norderstedt / Germany